# Eat Yourself Slim & Never Diet Again

## The 40-Day Plan That Will Transform Your Body and Mind Forever

Etrulia Reid Troy Lee, Ph.D.

All scripture quotations, unless otherwise indicated, are taken from the New King James Version®.
Copyright © 1982 by Thomas Nelson, Inc. Used by permission. All rights reserved.

All scriptures marked NIV are taken from the Holy Bible, New International Version®, NIV®.
Copyright © 1973, 1978, 1984, 2011 by Biblica, Inc.™ Used by permission of Zondervan. All
rights reserved worldwide. www.zondervan.com. The "NIV" and "New International Version" are
trademarks registered in the United States Patent and Trademark Office by Biblica, Inc.™

Scripture quotations marked NLT are taken from the Holy Bible, New Living Translation, copyright © 1996, 2004, 2007 by Tyndale House Foundation. Used by permission of Tyndale House
Publishers, Inc., Carol Stream, Illinois 60188. All rights reserved.

Scripture quotations from THE MESSAGE. Copyright © by Eugene H. Peterson 1993, 1994, 1995,
1996, 2000, 2001, 2002. Used by permission of NavPress Publishing Group.

**Disclaimer:** This publication is for informational purposes only. It is neither the intent of the author
or the publisher to render professional services to the reader. It is not intended to diagnose, treat,
cure, or prevent any health problem or condition. It is not intended to be a substitute for medical
advice. Always consult your physician or other health professional on matters regarding your health
and before embarking on any weight loss program. The author and publisher specifically disclaim
all responsibility for any liability, loss, injury, or risk, personal or otherwise, which is incurred as a
consequence, directly or indirectly, from the use or application of any contents in this book.

Any and all product names referred to in this publication are the trademarks of and property of their
respective owners. None of these owners has sponsored, authorized, endorsed or approved this publication in any way. The author received no financial remuneration for mentioning any products in
this publication. The statements made in this publication have not been evaluated by the Food and
Drug Administration of the United States of America.

ISBN-10: 1475033184
ISBN-13: 9781475033182

*Make your weight-loss journey more exciting at the*

*Eat Yourself Slim & Never Diet Again
Online Boot Camp!*

*Online six -week boot camps are powerful, energizing, and motivating to help you shake the weight for good! Designed to parallel your journey as you read this book, online sessions allow you to interact live with Dr. Troy every week, receive coaching, and pair up with an accountability partner. Go to* www.eatyourselfslimandneverdietagain.com *to register for the next session.*

# ACKNOWLEDGEMENTS

I thank my God and my Lord and Savior Jesus Christ, who gave me the skills, abilities, and passion to pursue this project.

I thank my husband of thirty-three years, Arvid Lee, who has always been the wind beneath my wings. Thank you for your encouragement, your support, and the belief that I would succeed at this. Your love for me continues to amaze me every day. I am blessed that you are my life partner and my love for you is without limits.

Thanks to my two wonderful sons Chay Lee and Michael Lee, for cheering me on as I toiled with this book. I admire the tenacity that you both possess in going for your dreams in life. You have made me one proud mama and I love you immensely.

With the love that only a mother and daughter can possess, share, and understand, I thank my mommy, Etrulia Lucille "Trudy" Reid, who has faced life's challenges with courage and tenacity, and who at eighty-five, is still looking forward to a glorious future. Trudy, I love you dearly.

I thank my sisters, Darlene Reid Ford, Patricia Reid Merritt, Jessica Reid Lanier, and Suzette Reid Royster, my brother, Alfred Reid, and my sister-aunt, Nita Chapel, for being perfect examples of setting goals and achieving them no matter what the obstacles. I cherish every moment that we spend together.

Thank you, Celeste Owens and Shirley Curry, for your guidance in the writing and editing of this book. I appreciate you for sharing your time and talent so generously with me.

Finally, I thank everyone who has ever listened to, applauded, learned from, tolerated, queried, or has just been dumbfounded with my ramblings about healthy eating and weight control. All of you have contributed in some way to my drive to write this book and I am grateful.

# TABLE OF CONTENTS

# Prologue

*What has trapped you in a body in a size that you do not want to be?*
*Who's to blame for your despair and at times your musings?*
*Is it Mickey D's quarter pounders that cause your weight to creep up,*
*Or the delightful Frappuccinos from Starbucks that you like to sup?*
*Are you too busy with so many things to do on your plate,*
*That the last thing on your mind is what's on your plate?*
*Morning breakfast consists of whatever you grab at the drive-thru,*
*Because you have to get to work early, you have so much to do.*
*Donut and coffee is your mid-morning pick-me-up sugar fix,*
*Could it be that is what is making your thighs so thick?*
*One too many office parties with colleagues' birthdays to celebrate,*
*Where you piled the goodies high on that tiny, little plate.*
*Skipping meals, making your metabolism slow down,*
*So when you get on the scale, like Flavor Flav you say, "Wow!!!"*
*However you got here, this is not where you want to stay,*
*And you have tired of saying, "I'll lose the weight one day."*
*Now is the best time on the planet for you to snatch your sexy back.*
*And you now have the tools to keep you on track.*
*You are ready to eat yourself slim, so you will never diet again.*
*Push off, embark, take the plunge—it is time to begin!*

# INTRODUCTION

Two frogs were sitting on the edge of a well. One frog decided to jump into the well. How many frogs were left on the edge of the well?

Did you answer one? Well, that would be an incorrect answer. The answer is two. Why? Because the one frog only decided to jump into the well, but he never did. He never took action.

How many times have you decided to lose weight? Did you actually do it? How many times have you been on a diet? How many times have you lost a few pounds only to gain them back again? How many pant sizes do you have in your closet? Do you have clothes in your closet that you have not worn in years, but you won't give them away because one day, someday, you will be that size again? Are you tired of playing these games with yourself?

If you can relate to the above questions and you do not feel good about your answers, then you will be happy that you picked up this book. This may be your kairos moment. The word kairos is a word that was used in ancient Greek times that means the right or opportune time for something to happen. It also carries with it the idea that if something is going to happen at this opportune time, it must be driven through with force.

If you are ready, it is time for you to use the force that exists within you to achieve the weight and body that you desire, that you deserve. If you will faithfully follow the plan in this book, you will have a new mindset in just forty days that will allow you to harness the power of your mind to not only transform your body, but to transform any area in your life.

Why forty days? Forty has special significance in the Bible as the time needed to prepare to step into a new season. Consider the following:

- It rained for forty days and forty nights when God destroyed the world with flooding water (Genesis 7:12).

- Moses was on the mountain with God for forty days and nights (Exodus 34:29).
- The children of Israel wandered in the desert for forty years (Exodus 16:35).
- Jesus fasted for forty days in the wilderness before beginning His ministry (Matthew 4:2).
- This is God's doing: A woman is pregnant 40 weeks!

While it is a generally accepted fact in psychology that it takes at least thirty days to practice a new habit before it becomes natural to you, the forty-day experiences in the Bible marked significant shifts in the order of things. The goal is for you to experience a significant shift in your eating habits such that your new habits will last for a lifetime!

This book will not only help you to transform your mind, it will also help you to transform your palate. As you begin to learn new information about what you eat and how it affects your body, your desire to destroy your body with unhealthy food will wane. As you gain a new appreciation for the awesome creation that you are, your desire to honor your body with healthy food will soar! I can't promise that you will never want a hot-fudge sundae again (I still eat them occasionally), but you will have a new desire to walk in a newness of life and thought.

*Eat Yourself Slim and Never Diet Again* is based on two factors: The first factor is learning to eat according to the principles outlined in the hunter-gatherer diet. The second factor is based on the latest findings on how to help people associate feelings of joy and excitement with weight loss rather than the traditional feelings of deprivation, pain, and hunger. Using powerful tools such as daily affirmations, prayers, visualization, songs, , and dream boards, participants stay motivated and happy as they take their joyous journey to a slim body.

As I pondered what to include and not include in this book, I reduced it down to the information that is essential for you to be successful in transforming your mind and your body. I wanted this book to be complete, without being too voluminous to read. As I tried to achieve this objective, I narrowed the essential information down to seven topics. When I looked at the topics of each chapter, I felt a sense of completeness. Then it struck me that the number seven was symbolic of completion in the Holy Bible. I thought, "Praise God!" I must be on the right path! If you are not familiar with the significance of the number seven in the Bible, here are just a few facts:

- God rested on the seventh day after he created the world (Genesis 2:2)
- In the Book of Revelation, there are seven churches, seven spirits, seven stars, seven seals, seven trumpets, seven vials, seven personages, seven dooms, and seven new things.
- There are seven days in a week.
- There are only seven musical notes; all notes are just a variation of the basic seven.

Seven is also the number of the letters in the word VICTORY. And in just seven chapters, you will have victory with a new mind and a new body!

There are more than 200 diets on the market today that promise to be the perfect fix for you to lose weight. You will be happy to know that I am not going to add another diet to the list. Rather, I am going to use known scientific principles of how to eat to be slim for life, which forms the basis for many popular diets today.

There are no prescribed meals in this book and no recipes. You get to choose what you eat, following certain nutritional principles. There are thousands of recipes online for you to choose from, and it was not my intention to add filler to this book, so I purposely left them out. However, I do give you some suggestions on what could make your meals more interesting.

Even with all the techniques that *Eat Yourself Slim and Never Diet Again* uses, the key to success is YOU. You must bring a readiness to change and an attitude that this is your time to change. So if you are ready to change, and this is your kairos moment where you are actually ready to DO rather than just decide, let's get started!

*Beloved, I pray that you may prosper in all things and be in health, just as your soul prospers.*
3 John 1:2 (NKJV)

# CHAPTER ONE
# WHY YOU WEIGH WHAT YOU WEIGH

*"As a man thinks in his heart, so is he."*
Proverbs 23:7 (NKJV)

*"It is the nature of thought to find its way into action."*
Christian Nevell Bovee

You weigh what you weigh because of one of three reasons:
1. You have an underlying medical condition such as hypothyroidism, metabolic syndrome, loss of mobility, etc., or have a medical condition that requires taking medications such as prednisone that cause weight gain.
2. Your beliefs about food and exercise cause you to think and act in a certain way.
3. You are uneducated about how food and exercise affects weight gain, which means you have some faulty beliefs.

Before embarking on any program to lose excess weight, it is recommended that you have a physical exam by your physician to rule out any medical concerns that may be the cause of your being overweight. Statistics are fuzzy, but it is estimated that less than 1 percent of people who are overweight have an underlying medical condition as the cause.

That would mean that you more than likely fall into the 99 percent category of people who are overweight because of your beliefs. You have a belief about food, your health, and exercise that causes you to think and act in a certain way. All actions in life are preceded by a thought. You think and then you act. You may have heard this quote before by Ralph Waldo Emerson:

> *"Sow a thought and you reap an action; sow an act and you reap a habit; sow a habit and you reap a character; sow a character and you reap a destiny."*

There have been thoughts sown in your mind about food, your health, and exercise that have caused you to reap a destiny of being overweight. Let's take a look at some possible beliefs that you hold and the origin of those beliefs.

## LEARNED BEHAVIOR FROM CHILDHOOD

Many of our thoughts about food stem from childhood. Maybe you had a parent who always told you to *"clean your plate; there are children starving in Africa,"* so you feel compelled to eat everything that is on your plate. This can be particularly troublesome in today's times when eating out at a restaurant where portion sizes are out of control.

### *Underlying belief: I must eat everything that is set before me.*

Maybe you had over-indulgent parents who did not know how to say "no" when it came to whatever you wanted to eat. As a result, you do not readily discipline yourself when it comes to what you eat.

### *Underlying belief: I do not need to discipline my eating habits.*

Did you suffer from food insecurity as a child? Food insecurity is a term used to describe a lack of access to food. A person has food insecurity when she is afraid she will go hungry and not have the resources to eat. I had food insecurity that stemmed from childhood that caused me to overeat whenever I was at an event where food was being served.

I am from a large family of nine children. We grew up in a nice, working-class neighborhood in Philadelphia. My mother worked very hard to provide our support, while my father—not so much. Although my mother worked, we were eligible for the surplus food program. The surplus food program was the government's program to help out needy families before the food stamp program was enacted. The embarrassing part of this program was that we had to go to the local recreation center with a wagon and pick up the food. Translation: everyone on the block—all sixty-three houses, knew that we were getting the surplus food. You can imagine the teasing!

I thank God that I did eat every day, but many of the meals lacked gourmet appeal, and loading up on seconds was not an option. I remember meals of beans and rice, other meals where chicken backs and necks were served (we could not afford more substantial parts of the chicken), and the one meal I hated the most was rice, spinach, and sardines. Ever eaten a mayonnaise sandwich? When there was nothing else to put on the bread but mayonnaise, you did what you had to do!

I was in my mid-thirties and was at an event, and believe or not, they were serving fish sticks. I remember being first or almost the first in line (this was a habit that I regularly practiced to make sure I would eat), and putting several fish sticks on my plate. I then remember going back for more fish sticks. As I sat eating my second serving of fish sticks, my inner voice said to me, *"Why are you eating these fish sticks? You don't even like them! You now earn enough money to eat lobster every night if you want to. This needs to stop."*

This was the start of a change of behavior in me towards food. The need to overeat at events became a thing of the past. Now if I overeat, which is rare, it is because I am chomping down on something way too delicious to avoid!

### *Underlying belief: I need to eat all the food I can while it is available.*

## ADVERTISING INFLUENCES

If your thoughts about food are not stemming from childhood habits, they are certainly influenced by the bombardment of TV, radio, Internet, and billboard advertising to eat unhealthy food. The Federal Trade Commission presented a report to Congress in July 2008 titled *Marketing Food to Children: A Review of Industry Expenditures, Activities and Self- Regulation.*

The report noted that the combined expenditures of forty-four companies on promotional activities for food and beverages were a whopping $9.6 billion. Companies make huge investments to separate you from your food dollars.

Think about the powerful images you see on TV when companies are advertising junk food: people smiling and having a good time, with lots of laughter; they always seem to be active; they have perfect hair and teeth, are slim and fit, are in a romantic relationship, and are oh so sexy! How many ads do you see of overweight people eating junk food? Nada!

And you know these slogans:

> Da-da-da-da-da...I'm loving it!
> Have a Coke and a smile
> Every Pepsi refreshes the world
> Think outside the bun
> It's waaaay better than fast food
> We do chicken right
> Love that chicken from Popeye's
> The king of beers
> The loudest taste on earth

Proverbs 4:23 tells us, *"Above all else, guard your heart, for everything you do flows from it."* (NIV). A key factor in guarding your heart is monitoring the influences you are being exposed to regularly. The amount of time that you see and hear TV and radio ads promoting unhealthy food influences what you eat. You cannot escape the billboards and the plethora of fast food outlets as you interact in the world nor the internet ads, but you can control what you allow in when you are in your home and in your car.

Be honest: how many times has a TV or radio commercial caused you to crave a food or a dining experience? You were not thinking about pizza until you saw the TV ad for the double-stuffed-crust-triple-meat pizza deal. The Chik-Fil-A commercial set off a desire for a milkshake that could be only quelled by you making a quick run to get one. The Madison Avenue wizards who create these commercials have us all trained like the Pavlov's dog: They advertise, we buy!

**_Underlying belief: I believe whatever the advertisers want me to believe._**

## ADDICTION TO PROCESSED FOODS

Ever wonder why you cannot duplicate the meal from your favorite restaurant or why your made-from-scratch hamburger and noodle casserole just does not taste the same as Hamburger Helper? That is because you do not have at your disposal the array of 3,000-plus chemical additives that the government has approved for use in foods. Food manufacturers mix and toss these additives with all the aplomb of a modern-day wizard, making food concoctions that send your taste buds into overdrive.

Consider the thirty-seven ingredients below and see if you can guess what food this is.

_Enriched Bleached Wheat Flour {Flour, Reduced Iron, B Vitamins (Niacin, Thiamine Mononitrate (B1), Riboflavin (B2), Folic Acid)}, Corn Syrup, Sugar, High Fructose Corn Syrup, Water, Partially Hydrogenated Vegetable and/or Animal Shortening (Soybean, Cottonseed and/or Canola Oil, Beef Fat), Whole Eggs, Dextrose. Contains 2% or Less of: Modified Corn Starch, Glucose, Leavenings (Sodium Acid Pyrophosphate, Baking Soda, Monocalcium Phosphate), Sweet Dairy Whey, Soy Protein Isolate, Calcium and Sodium Caseinate, Salt, Mono and Diglycerides, Polysorbate 60, Soy Lecithin, Soy Flour, Cornstarch, Cellulose Gum, Sodium Stearoyl Lactylate, Natural and Artificial Flavors, Sorbic Acid (to Retain Freshness), Yellow 5, Red 40._

The answer is listed at the end of the chapter. How many non-food additives did you count? What is modified cornstarch and how is it modified?

Check out this next food with thirty-four ingredients, brimming with not one, but three flavor enhancers to tickle your taste buds (flavor enhancers underlined), and then they throw in artificial flavors (how many?) to make the mystery of this food complete!

_Whole Corn, Vegetable Oil (Contains One or More of the Following: Corn, Soybean and/or Sunflower Oil), Corn Maltodextrin, Salt, Tomato Powder, Corn Starch, Lactose, Whey, Nonfat Milk, Corn Syrup Solids, Onion Powder, Sugar, Garlic Powder, <u>Monosodium Glutamate</u>, Cheddar_

*Cheese (Milk, Cheese Cultures, Salt, Enzymes), Dextrose, Malic Acid, Buttermilk, Natural and Artificial Flavors, Sodium Acetate, Artificial Color (Including Red 40, Blue 1, Yellow 5), Sodium Caseinate, Spice, Citric Acid, <u>Disodium Inosinate</u>, and <u>Disodium Guanylate</u>.*

Have you ever found yourself craving an apple the way you crave your favorite brand of soda or your favorite fast food? The answer is probably no. Dr. Michael Dow of the Sharecare community responds this way to the question of whether or not fast food is addictive:

*When you consider that a glass of wine and the amount of fat in a cheeseburger release about the same amount of dopamine in the brain, you can understand why both alcohol and fatty food can be addictive, so yes. In studies, we see the same withdrawal symptoms in rats given fatty food all the time just like rats given cocaine, so yes—it is {addictive}. Occasional exposure doesn't cause addiction with fast food. Think of it like tequila. Having a shot once in a while on a Friday night is fine for non-alcoholics, but if you had tequila with every meal, we have a problem.*

Processed food is created for shelf life, profit, and to keep you coming back for more since you cannot duplicate it at home. Our supermarkets and restaurants have become "drug pushers," with chemicals that are every bit as addictive as what you can find on the street corner.

### Underlying belief: I can eat processed foods regularly; it is OK and it is not harmful.

## SOCIETAL PRESSURES TO OVEREAT

We live in a society that is obsessed with food. It would be great if the food we were obsessed with was healthy, but it isn't; we live in a toxic food environment. Everywhere you turn, there are temptations to eat food that is unhealthy. Think of your average continental breakfast at a business meeting: Danish, bagels, donuts, coffee. Open house at your child's school: cookies and punch. Office birthday celebrations: cake. Sitting on the receptionist's desk: candy dish. What about just walking down the street and having your olfactory senses bombarded with an array of good smells? And what is it about the smell of bar-b-que or food frying that will derail all of our good intentions?

What happens when you are in a social setting and decide not to indulge? You are ridiculed. I have been made to feel like a monster with green horns more than once at work or at a party when my plate was not laden down with high-fat foods. Peer pressure does not only happen to children and to teens; it happens to adults as well. Our need to conform is driven by a basic need to be loved and accepted.

*Underlying belief: I must eat in social settings to be accepted and have a good time.*

## EMOTIONAL EATING

Emotional eating occurs when a person eats for a reason other than the fact that he is hungry. The reason he is eating could be because he is happy, sad, stressed, bored, anxious, etc. Here's a scene that sticks in my mind: once I was at a luncheon with some work colleagues, and after the meal, one of the ladies positioned her dessert in front of her and said, "Now it is time for me to have some fun!" Emotions of happiness and good times were clearly tied to her eating the dessert!

The experts at WebMD note the following differences in emotional eating versus physical hunger:

1. Emotional hunger comes on suddenly; physical hunger gradually.
2. When you are eating to fill a void that isn't related to an empty stomach, you crave a specific food, such as pizza or ice cream, and only that food will meet your need. When you eat because you are actually hungry, you're open to options.
3. Emotional hunger feels like it needs to be satisfied instantly with the food you crave; physical hunger can wait.
4. Even when you are full, if you are eating to satisfy an emotional need, you are more likely to keep eating. When you are eating because you are hungry, you are more likely to stop when you are full.
5. Emotional eating can leave behind feelings of guilt; eating when you are physically hungry does not.

If you believe that a deep-rooted emotional issue is the cause of your overeating, you may want to seek professional counseling so you can resolve any issues and gain better coping strategies. Also, it is important to note that emotional eating could be tied to food addiction in that certain foods release certain neurotransmitters in our brain that make us feel better.

### *Underlying belief: Food makes me feel better and is a part of my emotional well-being.*

## MINDLESS EATING

I am convinced that most of us are on a "see food" diet: we see food, we eat it! This is a result of bad habits rather than emotional issues. Brian Wansink in his book *Mindless Eating* notes:

> *Most of us don't overeat because we're hungry. We overeat because of family and friends, packages and plates, names and numbers, labels and lights, colors and candles, shapes and smells, distractions and distances, cupboards and containers. ... After conducting hundreds of food studies, I'm increasingly convinced that our stomach has only three settings: 1) We either feel like we're starving, 2) we feel like we're stuffed, or 3) we feel like we can eat more. Most of the time we're in the middle, we're neither hungry nor full, but if something's put in front of us, we'll eat it.*

### *Underlying belief: I see food, I eat it!*

Regardless of why we eat what we eat, we can all agree on one thing: Eating good food gives us enormous pleasure! God created us with taste buds to enjoy the bounty of the earth. Good food is tied to good times and family celebrations. The emotional memories surrounding food are real and are part of our cultural heritages. All of us have times of overindulgence and this is appropriate as we celebrate special occasions. Here's the problem: while I would agree that every day should be a celebration of life and we should live each as if it were our last, this should not extend to overindulging in food every day, and in unhealthy food at that. In order to be slim for life, we must learn to eat to live, rather than live to eat.

Now that we have examined some of the beliefs you may have about food, let's look at what you may believe about your health and exercise.

## BELIEFS ABOUT HEALTH

Not only do you have beliefs about food, you have a belief about your health. Sometimes I do not know whether to call this a belief or whether people are just in denial. According to the Centers for Disease Control, obesity lowers life expectancy and being overweight puts you at risk for developing a host of maladies. The major ones are highlighted below:

- Cancer
- Coronary heart disease
- Fatty liver disease
- Hypertension
- Gallbladder disease
- Metabolic syndrome
- Osteoarthritis
- Sleep apnea
- Type 2 diabetes

Let's look at the issue of cancer. According to the National Cancer Institute, a division of National Institutes of Health (NIH):

- A recent report estimated that in the United States, 14 percent of deaths from cancer in men and 20 percent of deaths in women were due to overweight and obesity.
- In 2001, experts concluded that cancers of the colon, breast (postmenopausal), endometrium (the lining of the uterus), kidney, and esophagus are associated with obesity. Some studies have also reported links between obesity and cancers of the gallbladder, ovaries, and pancreas.
- In 2002, about 41,000 new cases of cancer in the United States were estimated to be due to obesity.
- Weight gain during adulthood has been found to be the most consistent and strongest predictor of breast cancer risk in studies in which it has been examined.
- Overweight and obese individuals are two times more likely than healthy-weight people to develop a type of esophageal cancer called esophageal adenocarcinoma.
- Studies have consistently found a link between a type of kidney cancer (renal cell carcinoma) and obesity in women, with some studies finding risk among obese women to be two to four times the risk of women of a healthy weight.

- Obesity has been consistently associated with uterine (endometrial) cancer. Obese women have two to four times greater risk of developing the disease than do women of a healthy weight, regardless of menopausal status. Obesity has been estimated to account for about 40 percent of endometrial cancer cases in affluent societies.

If you are overweight and are ignoring the fact that you are putting your health at risk by carrying extra weight, this could be your underlying belief:

*I know of overweight people who are disease free, and I know people who were overweight and lived a long life. I will be like them. It won't get sick or die prematurely.*

## BELIEFS ABOUT EXERCISE

If you are not exercising regularly, and you are physically able to do so, there may be just one underlying belief.

*Exercise is not important to my health.*

## ASSESSING HEALTHY BODY WEIGHT

There are three ways to determine what a good body weight is for you and whether or not you need to lose weight. The first is to check your weight against a height and weight chart. Check your weight against the charts included on the next page.

A second way is to determine your body mass index (BMI). This measurement is based on your height and weight and is a good indicator of body fatness. You can calculate your BMI by looking at the chart included in this book or use an online calculator. A BMI calculator is located on our webpage at www.eatyourselfslimandneverdietagain.com.

## HEIGHT & WEIGHT CHART FOR WOMEN

| Height Feet Inches | Small Frame | Medium Frame | Large Frame |
|---|---|---|---|
| 4' 10" | 102-111 | 109-121 | 118-131 |
| 4' 11" | 103-113 | 111-123 | 120-134 |
| 5' 0" | 104-115 | 113-126 | 122-137 |
| 5' 1" | 106-118 | 115-129 | 125-140 |
| 5' 2" | 108-121 | 118-132 | 128-143 |
| 5' 3" | 111-124 | 121-135 | 131-147 |
| 5' 4" | 114-127 | 124-138 | 134-151 |
| 5' 5" | 117-130 | 127-141 | 137-155 |
| 5' 6" | 120-133 | 130-144 | 140-159 |
| 5' 7" | 123-136 | 133-147 | 143-163 |
| 5' 8" | 126-139 | 136-150 | 146-167 |
| 5' 9" | 129-142 | 139-153 | 149-170 |
| 5' 10" | 132-145 | 142-156 | 152-173 |
| 5' 11" | 135-148 | 145-159 | 155-176 |
| 6' 0" | 138-151 | 148-162 | 158-179 |

## HEIGHT & WEIGHT CHART FOR MEN

| Height Feet Inches | Small Frame | Medium Frame | Large Frame |
|---|---|---|---|
| 5' 2" | 128-134 | 131-141 | 138-150 |
| 5' 3" | 130-136 | 133-143 | 140-153 |
| 5" 4" | 132-138 | 135-145 | 142-156 |
| 5' 5" | 134-140 | 137-148 | 144-160 |
| 5' 6" | 136-142 | 139-151 | 146-164 |
| 5' 7" | 138-145 | 142-154 | 149-168 |
| 5' 8" | 140-148 | 145-157 | 152-172 |
| 5' 9" | 142-151 | 148-160 | 155-176 |
| 5' 10" | 144-154 | 151-163 | 158-180 |
| 5' 11" | 146-157 | 154-166 | 161-184 |
| 6' 0" | 149-160 | 157-170 | 164-188 |
| 6' 1" | 152-164 | 160-174 | 168-192 |
| 6' 2" | 155-168 | 164-178 | 172-197 |
| 6' 3" | 158-172 | 167-182 | 176-202 |
| 6' 4" | 162-176 | 171-187 | 181-207 |

## BODY MASS INDEX (BMI) CHART
Chart accessed at http://www.bmi-calculator.net/bmi-chart.php

| BMI | 19 | 20 | 21 | 22 | 23 | 24 | 25 | 26 | 27 | 28 | 29 | 30 | 35 | 40 |
|---|---|---|---|---|---|---|---|---|---|---|---|---|---|---|
| Height | Weight (lb.) | | | | | | | | | | | | | |
| 4'10" | 91 | 96 | 100 | 105 | 110 | 115 | 119 | 124 | 129 | 134 | 138 | 143 | 167 | 191 |
| 4'11" | 94 | 99 | 104 | 109 | 114 | 119 | 124 | 128 | 133 | 138 | 143 | 148 | 173 | 198 |
| 5'0" | 97 | 102 | 107 | 112 | 118 | 123 | 128 | 133 | 138 | 143 | 148 | 153 | 179 | 204 |
| 5'1" | 100 | 106 | 111 | 116 | 122 | 127 | 132 | 137 | 143 | 148 | 153 | 158 | 185 | 211 |
| 5'2" | 104 | 109 | 115 | 120 | 126 | 131 | 136 | 142 | 147 | 153 | 158 | 164 | 191 | 218 |
| 5'3" | 107 | 113 | 118 | 124 | 130 | 135 | 141 | 146 | 152 | 158 | 163 | 169 | 197 | 225 |
| 5'4" | 110 | 116 | 122 | 128 | 134 | 140 | 145 | 151 | 157 | 163 | 169 | 174 | 204 | 232 |
| 5'5" | 114 | 120 | 126 | 132 | 138 | 144 | 150 | 156 | 162 | 168 | 174 | 180 | 210 | 240 |
| 5'6" | 118 | 124 | 130 | 136 | 142 | 148 | 155 | 161 | 167 | 173 | 179 | 186 | 216 | 247 |
| 5'7" | 121 | 127 | 134 | 140 | 146 | 153 | 159 | 166 | 172 | 178 | 185 | 191 | 223 | 255 |
| 5'8" | 125 | 131 | 138 | 144 | 151 | 158 | 164 | 171 | 177 | 184 | 190 | 197 | 230 | 262 |
| 5'9" | 128 | 135 | 142 | 149 | 155 | 162 | 169 | 176 | 182 | 189 | 196 | 203 | 236 | 270 |
| 5'10" | 132 | 139 | 146 | 153 | 160 | 167 | 174 | 181 | 188 | 195 | 202 | 207 | 243 | 278 |
| 5'11" | 136 | 143 | 150 | 157 | 165 | 172 | 179 | 186 | 193 | 200 | 208 | 215 | 250 | 286 |
| 6'0" | 140 | 147 | 154 | 162 | 169 | 177 | 184 | 191 | 199 | 206 | 213 | 221 | 258 | 294 |
| 6'1" | 144 | 151 | 159 | 166 | 174 | 182 | 189 | 197 | 204 | 212 | 219 | 227 | 265 | 302 |
| 6'2" | 148 | 155 | 163 | 171 | 179 | 186 | 194 | 202 | 210 | 218 | 225 | 233 | 272 | 311 |
| 6'3" | 152 | 160 | 168 | 176 | 184 | 192 | 200 | 208 | 216 | 224 | 232 | 240 | 279 | 319 |
| 6'4" | 156 | 164 | 172 | 180 | 189 | 197 | 205 | 213 | 221 | 230 | 238 | 246 | 287 | 328 |

To use the chart, find your height on the left side of the page and then move across to find a weight that is closest to your weight. Then move your finger up the page to find your BMI.

- If your BMI is less than 18.5, it falls within the "underweight" range.
- If your BMI is 18.5 to 24.9, it falls within the "normal" or "healthy weight" range.
- If your BMI is 25.0 to 29.9, it falls within the "overweight" range.
- If your BMI is 30.0 or higher, it falls within the "obese" range.

The third way to determine if you need to lose weight is to measure your waist circumference. The medical community believes that belly fat is the most dangerous type to have because it is actually more biologically active than fat that settles in the hips, thighs, and buttocks. The fact that this fat is more biologically active results in calcium build-up in our arteries, which leads to heart attack and stroke. This is important because a person could have a normal BMI and be within the correct range for his height and weight, but still need to lose weight in his stomach area. According to

Dr. Gupta of CNN Health, a research study recently published in the *New England Journal of Medicine* found that people with belly fat have a higher risk of dying compared to their peers without a spare tire.

To measure your waist circumference, place a tape measure right above your hip bone. This should be right on if not very close to your belly button. Relax your mid-section. Place the tape measure around your waist so that it fits comfortably, but not too snug that your abdomen is protruding around the tape. If you are a woman, the measurement should be 35 inches or less, and if you are a man, the measurement should be 40 inches or less.

Now that you have taken the healthy weight assessment, you need to decide how much weight you want to lose and when you want to lose it. Please note this is not a program for you to get skinny. Fashion models are skinny and many are in fact underweight. Having a slim body means that you are within the ideal weight range and are not carrying excess belly fat. After all, the name of this book is *Eat Yourself Slim...*, not starve yourself skinny!

## EXERCISE ONE

## WHAT DO YOU WANT?

Now that you have invested your time and your money into this book, you need to get very clear about what it is you want from the program. In the space below, write out your weight loss goal.

How much weight do you want to lose? _____

_____

By what date would you like for this to occur? _____

_____

Why do you want to lose the weight? _____

_____
_____
_____
_____
_____
_____

Do you believe, or how do you believe, your life would be better when you achieve your weight loss goals? _____

_____
_____
_____
_____
_____
_____

Do you believe you have suffered from or missed anything in your life because of your weight? If yes, please describe. _____

_____
_____
_____
_____
_____
_____

## REFERENCES FOR CHAPTER ONE

Dow, M.. Accessed January 10, 2012 at http://www.sharecare.com/question/is-fast-food-really-addictive.

Gupta, S. *Is belly fat more dangerous for our health?* CNN Health. Accessed November 11, 2011 at http://thechart.blogs.cnn.com/2008/12/25/is-belly-fat-more-dangerous-to-our-health/

Hatfield, H. *Emotional eating: Feeding your feelings.* WebMD. Accessed November 5, 2011 http://www.webmd.com/diet/features/emotional-eating-feeding-your-feelings

Marketing Food to Children: *A Review of Industry Expenditures, Activities and Self- Regulation.* Accessed November 18, 2011 at http://www.ftc.gov/speeches/leibowitz/080729foodmarketingtochildren.pdf

National Cancer Institute. *Obesity and cancer: Questions and answers.* Accessed October 7, 2011 at http://www.cancer.gov/cancertopics/factsheet/Risk/obesity

Wansink, B. (2010). *Mindless eating: Why we eat more than we think.* New York: Bantam Books

Food #1: Twinkies

Food # 2: Cool Ranch Doritos

# CHAPTER TWO
## CHANGING YOUR MIND

*"Nobody can go back and start a new beginning, but anyone can start today and make a new ending."*
Maria Robinson

In order for any weight loss program to be successful, only three things must happen:

1. You must change your mind about the type and quantity of food you eat.
2. You must change your mind about exercise.
3. You must associate this change with joy and excitement.

Notice that the operative word is change. Since you have invested in this book, the assumption is that you are ready to be slim for life. But are you ready to make the change or were you just hoping for a magic potion or an easy way out? Before moving forward, it is important that you ask yourself the question, *"Am I ready to change?"*

In the study of the psychology of behavior change, there is what is known as the Transtheoretical Model of Change. This model proposes that there are five stages of change an individual goes through when behavior change occurs: precontemplation, contemplation, preparation, action, and maintenance.

The precontemplation stage is the stage in which there is no intention to change one's behavior. People in this stage are unaware that they have a problem or are aware that a problem exists but have no intention of changing their behavior.

In the contemplation stage, people are aware that a problem exists and are seriously thinking about doing something to correct the problem. However, they have not made a commitment to take action on the problem.

The preparation stage is where people prepare to make a change. People in this stage have a clear intention to take action and are preparing to take the action within thirty days or so.

The action stage is the stage in which people are deliberately taking action to change their behavior.

The maintenance stage is the stage in which people work to maintain the new behaviors that were implemented in the action stage. This stage will last for months or years, until the new behavior is so ingrained that it is automatic.

Which stage do you believe you are in right now? By reading this book, it is hoped that you are minimally in the contemplation stage and that you have taken this action to move into the preparation stage. But are you ready to take the action to change your behavior?

I am sure you have heard that change is hard. Leading experts offer a variety of reasons why this is so. One reason is that people fear the unknown. Since no one has a crystal ball to see into the future, we resist doing things from which we cannot be sure of the outcome.

Change stretches us to behave in a different manner from what we are used to. It stretches us outside of our familiar comfort zone. Many people want the comfort of what they know.

Change is also unpopular at times. The idea of "why fix it if it ain't broke" is the underlying refrain. Resistance to change is universal and it often invites animosity and tension.

Numerous research studies have been conducted on the contributing factors that get people to change their lifestyle from an unhealthy one to a healthy one. Most programs aimed at helping people live healthier lives provide people with knowledge, with the underlying belief that knowledge will change people's behavior. One scripture often quoted when people are attempting to educate others on a topic is Hosea 4:6:

*My people are destroyed for lack of knowledge.*

Somehow, everyone forgets to quote the rest of the verse:

*Because you have rejected knowledge, I also will reject you from being priest for Me; Because you have forgotten the law of your God, I also will forget your children. (NKJV)*

It is not that people _lack_ the knowledge of how to live a healthy lifestyle, people are _rejecting_ the knowledge. Embracing the knowledge and acting on the knowledge would lead to change in behavior, and many people do not want to change.

It has been said that "knowledge is power." This is probably one of the biggest untruths that has been quoted throughout history. Knowledge by itself is not power; it is what you do with knowledge that is power. And in this age of instant information via the Internet, we need to go a step further and say that what you do with *accurate* knowledge is power.

It is easy to believe that if a person knew life was in jeopardy because of an unhealthy lifestyle that would be sufficient to bring about a change in behavior. This is not true. It has been shown that even people who are at risk of death if they do not change their unhealthy lifestyle do not always change. An amazing example of this can be seen in people with coronary artery disease. Deutschman (2005) reports the following:

*Dr. Edward Miller, the dean of the medical school at Johns Hopkins University, reported that: "It is a well-documented fact that every year, about 600,000 people in the U.S. who have severe heart disease have bypass surgery and about 1.3 million heart patients have angioplasties." Angioplasty is a procedure used to open blocked or narrowed coronary arteries. Using a device called a stent, the procedure improves blood flow to the heart muscle and temporarily relieves chest pains, but they are not known to prevent heart attacks or extend a person's life. Around half of the time, the bypass grafts clog up in a few years; the angioplasties, in a few months. The causes of this so-called restenosis are complex. It's sometimes a reaction to the trauma of the surgery itself. But many patients could avoid the return of pain and the need to repeat the surgery—not to mention arrest the course of their disease before it kills them— by switching to healthier lifestyles. Yet very few do. "If you look at people after coronary-artery bypass grafting two years later, 90% of them have not changed their lifestyle," Miller said. "And that's been studied over and over and over again. And so we're missing some link in there. Even though they know they have a very bad disease and they know they should change their lifestyle, for whatever reason, they can't."*

*Considerable research has been aimed at identifying factors that contribute to successful lifestyle change and what it takes to help people adopt healthier habits. One problem may be that we're motivated too often by a sense of guilt, fear, or regret. Experts who study behavior change agree that long-lasting change is most likely when it's self-motivated and rooted in positive thinking. In October 2006, the Economic and Social Research Council, a British research group, released findings on 129 different studies of behavior change strategies. The survey confirmed that the least effective strategies were those that aroused fear or regret in the person attempting to make a change.*

Fear often grips a person when they thinking about dieting and changing their eating habits. Ever consider the word "diet?" What do the first three letters of the word spell? Die! And that is exactly what most people think is going to happen to them if they change their eating habits! We associate pain and deprivation with weight loss and healthy eating. As long as this is a person's mindset toward shedding unwanted pounds, weight loss is impossible.

Change is not impossible, but it does take effort. People do change, take risks, and engage in endeavors for which they are not sure of the outcome. Take the example of anyone who enters a romantic relationship. Talk about risks! People get married, combine their resources, move across the country, and start a new life together. People change and launch out on their own in business, not having any certainty of the outcome. When you consider these changes, you will note that people are making these changes at a time when they are joyful and excited about what the future will hold for them.

My goal is to help you change your mind about the food you are eating, and to help you get excited about changing your mind and your habits. Just like a newlywed couple or the new entrepreneur who are willing to take risks and change because they believe that their actions will lead to a better life, you must get excited and believe that the actions you are getting ready to take to transform your body is exciting and you anticipate a great outcome.

## YOUR BELIEFS

People know a lot of things, especially when it comes to truisms that are supposed to lead to a happy, healthy life. Such things as:

- Get plenty of rest
- Drink at least 8 glasses of water a day
- Exercise regularly
- Eat plenty of fruits and vegetables
- Avoid fried foods
- Cut down on desserts and sweets
- Don't smoke
- Do not take drugs (as opposed to doctor prescribed medication, which we hope is safe)

While people know these things to be true, they do not practice them. Humans by and large do not willingly set themselves up for pain, disease, and premature death. So why do people engage in behaviors that do not promote and protect their health?

They engage in these behaviors because they do not believe that anything untoward will happen to them. They know of people who smoked, took drugs, did not exercise, etc., and they lived to be a decent age in relatively good health. So they assume that they too can engage in risky health behaviors and have a good outcome.

Research tells us that knowing factual information is not enough to change a person's behavior. People do not act on what they know; they act on what they believe. And even when people believe something to be true, they may have a hard time changing their behavior to fit their new belief.

Right now as you sit reading this text, you have a belief about your weight. Inherent in that belief about your weight are beliefs regarding what is a good meal, a good time, healthy food, dieting, exercise, beverages, relaxation, etc. All of these beliefs are part of why you currently weigh what you do.

## EXERCISE TWO

As best as you honestly can, answer what you believe about each item. Do not think hard about this exercise. Just write the first thought that comes to your mind. The first thought you have is more than likely the truth about what you feel and what you believe.

People who are slender ... _____

_____

_____

Eating healthy food... _____

_____

_____

My idea of a good time is... _____

_____

_____

Drinking water..._____

_____

_____

Exercise is..._____

_____

_____

In order to lose weight... _____

_____

_____

I weigh what I currently weigh because... _____

_____

_____

In looking back over your answers, will the ideas/beliefs that you wrote down help you or hinder you on your journey to be slim? Go back and read over your answers and write the word "help" or "hinder" in the margin.

## EXERCISE THREE

In the spaces below, write down ten things you believe it will take for you to lose weight for good.

1. _____
   _____

2. _____
   _____

3. _____
   _____

4. _____
   _____

5. _____
   _____

6. _____
   _____

7. _____
   _____

8. _____
   _____

9. _____
   _____

10. _____
    _____

Now look at each belief in exercises two and three. If it is already an affirming belief that will encourage you on your journey to weight loss, great! We will keep that in our arsenal. If it is not a positive belief, use the space below to write the opposite of the negative belief. For example, if you wrote, "Losing weight is hard," replace that statement below with "Losing weight is easy with the right mindset."

1. _____
   _____

2. _____
   _____

3. _____
   _____

4. _____
   _____

5. _____
   _____

6. _____
   _____

7. _____
   _____

8. _____
   _____

9. _____
   _____

10. _____
    _____

Congratulations! You have just completed the first step towards changing your mind and enlisting it in helping you to be successful on your joyful journey of weight loss.

Your next step is to drill these new beliefs down into your spirit. Using 3 x 5 index cards, write down the new statements. When I am establishing a new belief, I use 3 x 5 cards that have been cut in half so I can fit them neatly in my purse or pocket. Your goal is to look at your new beliefs and say them out loud with enthusiasm every morning when you first wake up and every evening before you go to bed at night. You must do this at a bare minimum for the next thirty days. Why thirty days? It is a generally accepted fact in psychology that it takes at least thirty days of doing something for change to occur. This is true for new beliefs to take hold as well. In addition to your statements above, add these statements below:

I eat foods that build up my body.

I love fresh fruits and vegetables.

I am slender.

I am enjoying my weight reduction journey.

My slim body is emerging day by day.

I am a winner.

I can do whatever I set my mind to do.

My mind is made up and I am eating to be slim forever.

This new healthy way of eating is wonderful!

I am so proud of myself!

I am loving eating to be slim.

Eating to be slim is pure joy!

I am excited every morning when I wake up so I can be successful one more day in my new lifestyle of eating to be slim.

Eating to be slim is so much fun!

I giggle and give myself a high-five every night for how successful I was today at my new attitude towards healthy food.

I only spend my hard-earned money on food that is good for my body.

I easily pass up junk food.

I feel empowered when I eat the right things for my slim body.

Nothing tastes as good as being slim feels.

Notice that all of the statements above are in the affirmative, hence the word affirmations. If you choose to add additional statements, make sure they are stated in positive terms. Do not use statements about what you do not want; only what you want. For example, you would not say, "I am losing weight because I do not want to have heart disease," or "I am tired of not being able to walk up a flight of stairs without breathing hard."

## SING YOUR WAY SLIM

When is it that most people sing? They sing when they are happy and upbeat. And if someone is not happy before they start to sing, they will feel better after they start to sing. Julia Layton tells us the following about singing:

> Singing can have some of the same effects as exercise, like the release of endorphins, which give the singer an overall "lifted" feeling and are associated with stress reduction. It's also an aerobic activity, meaning it gets more oxygen into the blood for better circulation, which tends to promote a good mood. And singing necessitates deep breathing, another anxiety reducer. Deep breathing is a key to meditation and other relaxation techniques, and you can't sing well without it.

Singing is a powerful way to drive the message into your subconscious that you are eating yourself slim. This is a must-do step and cannot be skipped if you expect to have success with the program. Sing these tunes in the shower, while you are driving in your car, fixing dinner, etc. The tunes to all of the songs below can be found at www.eatyourselfslimandneverdietagain.com.

I've Got My Mind Made Up (To the tune *I've Got My Mind Made Up* by Donny McClurkin).

> I've got my mind made up, and I will move forth
> Cause I want to see my waistline real soon.
> I've got my mind made up, and I will move forth
> Cause I want to see my waistline real soon.
> Reducing carbs, I only eat small amounts.
> Reducing sweetened drinks, I rarely drink them at all.
> I've made up my mind, to eat to be slim, the rest of my life.
> I've made up my mind, to eat to be slim, the rest of my life.

I'm So Excited (To the tune of *I'm So Excited* by the Pointer Sisters).

> I'm so excited, and I just can't hide it.
> My body is getting slim and I think I like it.
> I'm so excited, and I just can't hide it.
> I'm about to shake the weight and I think I like it.

Got A New Way of Eating (Copyright © 2012)

Got a new way of eating, and my body likes it.

Fat is melting away; I'm getting slimmer every day. When I get on the scale, I like just what I see.

Numbers steady decreasing, there's so much less of me!

Closing in on 160, I'm locked and fully loaded.

Ready, aim, shoot bang, bang! I'm looking good and I know it.

Moving on to 150, I've got you in my sight.

Will be there by March 1st, and it feels soooo right.

(Use your own weight and date goal).

I've Got This Thing (Copyright © 2012)

I've got this thing, I'm in control.

Got my mind made up and I'm ready to roll!

I'm eating healthy, I'm feeling alright.

My body's slimming down, I'm looking pretty tight!

Haters, haters, you've got something to say,

Cause I'm passing on the sweets, get out of my way!

You wish you could rock this and be like me,

Just get off the couch and put down the cheese.

This is about me now, and it's about time.

Snatching back my sexy, my life is sublime!

Ain't No Stoppin Us Now

The lyrics in this song are virtually unchanged from the tune "Ain't No Stoppin Us Now" by McFadden and Whitehead.

Ain't no stoppin' me now

I'm on the move

Ain't no stopping me now

I've got my grove

There've been so many things that's held me down

But now I'm in control and things are turning around

I really don't have that far to go

And where I'll end up...I do know

Cause I won't let nothing hold me back

I've got myself together, gonna polish up my act

And I know I've been overweight before
But I refuse to be overweight anymore.
I won't let nothing, nothing, stand in my way.
I want you to listen, listen to every word I say,
Every word I say.
Ain't no stopping me now, I'm on the move.
Ain't no stopping me now, I'm on the move.

## PREPARE FOR YOUR HATERS

Not everybody will be happy and excited for you that you are losing weight. These people are called dream stealers and will do minor and major things to keep you from succeeding. Remember that people like the status quo and do not want you to change. Your change will make them feel uncomfortable because deep inside, they know they need to change as well.

Overweight people are in the majority in the United States, with about 68 percent of the population of adults age 20 and over being overweight or obese. Having the goal to be slimmer is going against the norm.

This question I want to ask you as gently as possible: Who are the people you hang around with? It has been said that we become like the people we associate with.  Researchers from Arizona State University's School of Human Evolution and Social Change in the U.S. in a study that involved over 100 women and their closest friends found that  the fatter a woman's social circle, the more likely she was to be obese herself.   If by choice most of your associates are overweight, then you may need to make some new friends. I am not saying to totally ditch your old friends, but you want to spend time with people who can encourage you in what you are doing, rather than derailing your efforts.

So let's get ready for your haters!

## EXERCISE FOUR

Who is it who will question the sanity of what you are doing?  _____

_____

_____

Think of some of the things that they may say to you. Prepare your answers in advance so you will be ready to disarm them so your weight loss efforts will not be sabotaged.

I have given you a few examples to start:

When they say: *Are you dieting again?*

You will say: *No, I am not dieting. But I am enjoying some new eating habits.*

When they say: *Oh, c'mon, it is Sally's birthday. Aren't you at least going to have some cake?*

You will say: *I'll pass on the cake. I find that my mind is clearer without all the sugar.*

Notice that each time you are saying out loud something positive about your new eating habits. You are not simply saying "no" or "no thank-you"; you are affirming your new behavior as being a good thing!

When they say: _____

_____

_____

You will say: _____

_____

_____

_____

When they say: _____

_____

_____

You will say: _____

_____

_____

When they say: _____

_____

_____

You will say: _____

_____

_____

## PREPARE FOR YOUR CHALLENGES

## EXERCISE FIVE

What challenges to your new eating plan will you encounter this week? Will it be an office lunch, a party, or a visit to a relative or friend who will insist on force-feeding you? Think in advance how you will handle the situation. You may refer to Chapter Seven for some insight into how to handle social situations. This is an activity you should engage in weekly. Having a plan in advance beats willpower every time!

Your plan for your challenges this week. _____

_____

_____

_____

_____

_____

_____

## THE SUCCESSFUL YOU

You are a successful person. You have the ability to achieve whatever you decide to achieve, providing it is not impossible. What are some of things that may be impossible for you to achieve?

> Being a top fashion model where the height requirement is 5'9" and above and you are 4'11".
> Deciding at sixty that you want a career as a ballerina.
> Wanting to be the fastest runner in the world and you have mobility issues.

O.K., you get the point. The real point is that what most people want to achieve, especially when it comes to their weight, eating healthy, improved financial health, better relationships with their loved ones, an increase in their competitive edge in the job market, starting their own business, etc. is achievable.

Think back over your life and consider some of the things that you have already achieved. How did you achieve them? Did you just wish them to be true, or did you put in some effort to make it happen? Your past successes are proof of your ability to achieve whatever you set your mind to achieve. It may have been a while since you achieved anything that you consider great or worthy of celebration, but at some point in your life you did. Remembering those past successes will help spur you on to achieve the success you are now seeking in having a slim body.

## EXERCISE SIX

Take a moment to reflect on some of things you have achieved in life that make you proud. I am not talking about having a prideful spirit. We all have something in life that we are proud of and we remember the great feeling of accomplishment when we achieved a certain task. It could be that you hit the winning run for your baseball team, had the leading role in a school play, won a science fair award, completed a certificate of training, got your GED, completed a college degree, won a seat on the student council, bought your first home after saving to do so, got out of debt, etc.

In the space that follows or on a separate sheet of paper, list all of the achievements that you can think of that bring you thoughts of pleasure and satisfaction. Key words: *list all.* Do not stop at just one or two. Really take time to think and reflect. Do not rush through this activity. You may want to grab a cup of warm tea or other relaxing drink and take your time to think about this. Let your mind wander and reflect on the successes of your life.

_____

_____

_____

_____

_____

_____

_____

_____

_____

_____

_____

_____

_____

_____
_____
_____
_____
_____
_____
_____
_____
_____
_____
_____
_____
_____
_____
_____
_____
_____
_____
_____
_____

Pick one of the events that you have on your list. You may do this activity immediately after you have made your list, or you may set aside another time for it when you have at least fifteen minutes to do the activity. Settle your mind and take a few deep breaths. Picture the event in your mind. Recall the exact moment when the success was officially declared. Recall all of the events that led up to the moment. Who was there? What did you wear? Where was the event held? What was the weather like? What time of year was it? Were there any special scents in the air? Recall everything about the event that you can. Visualize it as clearly in your mind as you can. Take your time enjoying your memories of how you felt before the event, at the event, and after the event.

Continue the above exercise until you have relived and visualized all of your successes. Do one a day until you have enjoyed all of the sweet, wonderful memories of the unstoppable you.

As you continue on your journey to the slim body that you want, if any doubts creep in that you will achieve your goal, remind yourself that you are a winner by remembering your past successes. Even better, if you have photos, awards, ribbons, plaques, etc. of your past achievements, dust them off and display them in a place where they can serve as daily reminders of the successful you. Allow yourself to relive the moments whenever you need to. This is the proof that the successful you is still there…it just needs a little coaxing to come out again.

## REFERENCES FOR CHAPTER TWO

Deutschman, A. *Change or die.* Accessed January 24, 2011 at http://www. fastcompany.com/magazine/94/open_change-or-die.html

Hruschka, D.J., Brewis, A.A., Wutich, A., Morin, B. (2011) *Shared norms and their explanation for the social clustering of obesity.* American Journal of Public Health[Electronic version]. Dec; 101 Suppl 1:S295-300.

Layton, J. *Does singing make you happy?* Accessed January 23, 2012 at http://health.howstuffworks.com/mental-health/human-nature/happiness/singing-happy1.htm

Prochaska, J.O., Velicer, W.F. (1997). *The Transtheoritical Model of Behavior Change. American Journal of Health Promotion.* Vol 12, pp. 38-48.

# CHAPTER THREE
## NUTRITION 101

This was the hardest section of this book for me write. I wanted to tell you everything that I knew! Having studied holistic nutrition I so desperately wanted to do a brain dump and tell you all of the evils of certain foods and the outrageous benefits of others. However, doing so would make this book much too long so I exercised restraint for your benefit. Instead of a brain dump I am going back to the principle of seven and will stick with what I believe are the seven most important things for you to know.

### POINT #1: YOUR BODY MAY BE ON FIRE!

Medical and health experts everywhere are sounding the alarm about the dangers of whole-body inflammation. Whole-body inflammation is now thought to be the culprit of a host of diseases in the body including cancer, heart disease, Alzheimer's, lupus, depression, Parkinson's, fibromyalgia, and multiple sclerosis just to name a few. Knowing the level of inflammation in your body and correcting it is key to your health, and it can be corrected with healthy eating.

When your body suffers an injury or is attacked by invaders such as germs, inflammation occurs in the body. Inflammation is the body's normal response to these threats. This inflammatory response helps the body mount immune defenses in the area where they are needed so the infection can be healed. However, this inflammatory response can go awry if it is not turned off when the body has healed. This is the case in autoimmune diseases like lupus, multiple sclerosis, and Crohn's disease.

Whole-body inflammation refers to low-level inflammation that is chronic and undiagnosed. This type of inflammation is thought to be due to lack of exercise, processed foods, and environmental toxins such as tobacco. In addition, excess body fat—especially abdominal fat— is believed to produce many substances that lead to inflammation in the body.

How do you know if you have chronic inflammation in your body? A simple blood test that can be done at the same time you have your annual blood work can measure inflammation. The name of the test is C-reactive protein (CRP). Believe it or not, most doctors rarely if ever order this test on a routine basis. I have been requesting it for the past eight years and monitoring my levels to make sure they are in the appropriate range. A healthy range for CRP is 0.00–3.00 mg/L. Any number above 3.0 means your body is in state of inflammation and you should take immediate steps to reduce it.

A while ago, I encouraged my husband to have his CRP level checked. As is the norm, he had to ask his doctor to include it in his lab work. His value came back at 9.7 mg/L. Do you think his physician said anything about his elevated levels? Not a word. What I was even more outraged at was that someone from the doctor's office gave him the report over the phone, so at least one person should have known that this was not good.

It so happened that I was seeing my cardiologist the next week. I told her about my husband's CRP value and she responded with "Woo, that is not good. He needs to get on top of that immediately." Needless to say, we booked an appointment for him with her right away!

I urge you to have your CRP level checked immediately. This is a marker of how healthy your body is and whether or not you are at risk for chronic disease. In addition, start adding as many anti-inflammatory foods to your meal plans as possible. An anti-inflammatory diet is one that includes lots of fresh fruits and vegetables, whole grains, and omega-3 fatty acids.

The website Nutrition Data at http://nutritiondata.self.com has a rating scale for most common foods. Some foods are inflammatory, while others are anti-inflammatory. A food that is inflammatory is given a negative rating while a food that is anti-inflammatory is given a plus rating. According to Nutrition Data, the goal is to balance negative foods with positive foods so that the combined rating for all foods eaten in a single day is positive with a net rating of +50.

## Some Common Foods' Inflammation Ratings
### Per Nutrition Data http://nutritiondata.self.com

| FOOD | SERVING SIZE | INFLAMMATION RATING |
|---|---|---|
| Whole wheat bread | 1 slice | -28 |
| White bread | 1 slice | -50 |
| French bread | 1 medium | -67 |
| Biscuits | 6 ounces | -95 |
| Yogurt, fruit, low fat | 1 cup | -115 |
| Low-fat 1% Milk | 1 ounce | -64 |
| Cheddar cheese | 1 whole | -26 |
| Egg | 1 cup | -174 |
| Brown rice | 1 medium | -143 |
| Baked white potato | 1 medium | -78 |
| Baked sweet potato | 1 cup | +216 |
| Black beans | 1 cup cooked | -45 |
| Kale | 1 cup shredded ` | +226 |
| Romaine lettuce | ½ cup shredded, cooked | +75 |
| Cabbage | 1 cup | +23 |
| String beans | 1 medium | +3 |
| Apple | 1 cup | -30 |
| Grapes | 1 large | -33 |
| Orange | 1 cup | +9 |
| Papaya | 1 ounce | +33 |
| Carrots | 1 small whole | +37 |
| Tomato | 1 ounce | +8 |
| Avocado | ½ breast, no skin | +22 |
| Chicken, roasted | ½ breast, skin | -18 |
| Chicken, fried | 3 ounces, no visible fat | -41 |
| Beef roast | 3 ounces steamed | +15 |
| Shrimp | 3 ounces | +140 |
| Salmon, Atlantic wild | 3 ounces | +494 |
| Tuna, light canned in water | 1 tablespoon | +138 |
| Olive oil | 1 ounce | +71 |
| Walnuts | 1 ounce | -38 |
| Almonds, raw | 1 ounce | +51 |
| Peanuts, dry roasted | 1 ounce | +19 |

## POINT #2: YOU ARE DESTROYING YOUR HEART AND BRAIN WITH THE WRONG TYPE OF FAT

When it comes to your diet, all fats are not created equal. It is kind of like in *The Wizard of Oz* where you had the good witch and the bad witch—the good fats help to protect your life, the bad fats help to destroy it.

*Saturated Fat*

Animal fat is a saturated fat. Meat, poultry, eggs, butter, cheese, and whole milk products are all saturated fats. Coconut oil and palm oil are also saturated fats.

For years, the conventional wisdom from medical professionals has been to eat a diet low in saturated fat to reduce your risk of heart disease. As of this writing, some holistic health professionals are rethinking their position because of recent studies that have shed new light on saturated fat and heart disease. Dr. Andrew Weil, world-renowned physician turned holistic health guru and a frequent guest on the Dr. Oz show, notes this in a recent post:

> *...My thinking on saturated fat has evolved. One catalyst was a scientific analysis of 21 earlier studies, which showed "no significant evidence" that saturated fat in the diet is associated with an increased risk of coronary heart disease. The 21 studies analyzed included nearly 348,000 participants, most of whom were healthy when they were enrolled. They were followed for five to 23 years, during which 11,000 developed heart disease or had a stroke. Looking back at the dietary information collected from these thousands of participants, the investigators found no difference in the risk of coronary heart disease, stroke, or coronary vascular disease between those individuals with the lowest and highest intakes of saturated fat. This goes completely against the conventional medical wisdom of the past 40 years. It now appears that many studies used to support the low-fat recommendation had serious flaws.*
>
> *In the meantime, as nutritionists have been recommending low-fat foods, consumption of added sweeteners, especially high-fructose corn syrup, has been steadily rising. This may be at least partially due to the fact that low-fat prepared foods are often highly sweetened. A study from Emory University and the U.S. Centers for Disease Control and Prevention*

*published in April, 2010, showed that sweeteners appear to lower levels of HDL ("good") cholesterol and raise triglycerides. Both of these effects increase the risk of heart disease. What's more, through their direct effects on insulin and blood sugar, refined starches and sugars are more likely than saturated fat to be the main dietary cause of coronary heart disease and type-2 diabetes.*

*...Given the results of these studies, I no longer recommend choosing low-fat dairy products. I believe the healthier choice is high quality, organic dairy foods in moderation. My personal choice would be high quality, natural cheese a few times a week. I don't advise eating saturated fat with abandon, because the foods that are full of it (salty bacon, conventionally raised beef, processed cheese) are often not the best for our health. Try to limit it to about ten percent of daily calories. You may choose to use your "budget" of saturated fat calories on ice cream, butter or high-quality natural cheese, or even an occasional steak (from organic, grass-fed, grass-finished cattle, please). I still recommended skinless chicken and turkey because poultry fat (concentrated just beneath the skin) contains arachidonic acid, which promotes inflammation. I also still recommend strictly avoiding foods that contain chemically altered fats (such as hydrogenated vegetable oils found in many prepared foods), as these do appear to raise cardiovascular disease risk.*

Before you begin to eat saturated fat with abandon, keep in mind that Dr. Weil is recommending that no more than 10 percent of your daily diet come from saturated fat. For most people, 10 percent of their daily calories from saturated fat amounts to 20 to 25 grams of saturated fat per day. The main point here is that if you choose, you can eat whole-fat products without feeling guilty, but they still should make up a very small portion of your diet.

The dangers of saturated fat as it relates to heart health have long been on the radar screen of health professionals. However, how saturated fat is affecting the brain is not being discussed. Carper (2000) states:

*"The type of fat you put in your brain from birth to death is one of the most critical decisions you can ever make for the good or detriment of your brain."*

Regarding saturated fats and the brain, The Franklin Institute Resources for Science and Learning reports studies have shown that:

- Animals fed lots of saturated fat don't learn as quickly or perform as well on memory tests.
- Animal studies show fetuses fed high-saturated-fat diets showed fewer and shorter dendrites (dendrites are extensions from brain cells {neurons} that are involved in the transmission of information from one brain cell to another).
- High–saturated-fat diets are associated with degenerative brain diseases such as Parkinson's and Alzheimer's
- Saturated fat degrades memory and learning by affecting the hormone insulin.

### Trans Fat

Trans fat (also called trans fatty acid) is a fat such as corn oil and soybean oil that is normally liquid at room temperature in its natural state, but is changed into a solid at room temperature when it is combined with hydrogen through a chemical process. These trans fats are called hydrogenated oil or partially hydrogenated oil. Any fat we eat that is liquid when heated but then turns into a solid when cooled to room temperature is either a saturated or trans fat. Margarines and Crisco are examples of trans fats. Also, any oil that is heated to a high temperature such as that required to fry food turns into a trans fat.

Trans fats, like saturated fats, are bad for your heart and arteries because they alter basic metabolic pathways, causing a rise in your bad (LDL) cholesterol levels, while causing a decrease in your good (HDL) levels. Trans fat also increases triglycerides, a type of fat found in your blood, which may contribute to hardening of the arteries. Hardening of the arteries increases the risk of stroke, diabetes, heart attack and heart disease.

Trans fat are also believed to increase inflammation in the body. We have already covered the dangers of inflammation previously in this chapter.

The havoc that trans fats are wreaking on your brain is startling. The Franklin Institute Resources for Science and Learning states:

> The human brain now faces a challenge never before encountered in its thousands of generations of development. During the past century, something has become fundamentally different with many of the fats we now consume. Modern food processing techniques have actually altered a basic building block of the brain. And not for the better.

*Trans fatty acids found in foods like French fries, margarine, potato chips and anything else with partially hydrogenated oil disrupt communication in your brain. Trans fatty acids are rarely found in nature and are mostly man made.*

*By modifying natural fats, we have altered the basic building blocks of the human brain—weakening the brain's architecture. And, like unstable buildings that come apart in an earthquake or storm, poorly structured human brains are failing to cope with the mounting stress of modern life.*

*Studies show that the trans fatty acids we eat do get incorporated into the brain cell membranes, including the myelin sheath that insulates the neurons. They replace the natural DHA in the membrane, and affect the electrical activity of the neuron. Trans fatty acid molecules disrupt communication, setting the stage for cellular degeneration and diminished mental performance.*

*Normal fatty acids have a natural curve to their molecular shape. When they fit together in vast numbers, enough space still remains so that the membrane has the proper structure it needs to function at its best. However, if these same fat molecules are changed by manufactured food processes, or if they are heated for long periods—as in deep-frying—they mutate into a form rarely found in nature. Now their molecules are straighter, narrower, and no longer have their original curved shape. This means that these altered fats will pack more tightly together into the cell membrane, making it more saturated and rigid—less flexible and less able to function properly. These altered fats are finally being recognized for the damage they cause. For half a century, however, hardly any attention was paid to them.*

Manufacturers of processed food prefer hydrogenated oils in their products because it increases shelf life. The government now requires that food manufacturers inform you on the label as to the amount of trans fat that food contains, but the government gave food manufacturers a loophole. If a product contains less than ½ (0.5) gram of trans fat per serving, the label can say that it has zero grams of trans fat. Here's the problem: most people do not eat one serving size, and they end up eating more trans-fat than they realize. So even if a label says a product has zero grams of trans fat, read the ingredient list. If you see hydrogenated or partially hydrogenated oil in the list of ingredients, it contains trans fat and is detrimental to your health.

The government recommends that you eat no more than 2 percent of your daily calories from trans fat, which is two grams. But the American Heart Association reports that in 2002, the government agreed with researchers for the first time on record stating that there is likely no safe level of trans fat in the diet and that people should eat as little as possible. Most holistic health professionals recommend that you totally avoid trans fat.

Avoiding trans fat requires a conscious effort, as they are ubiquitous. Here is just a brief partial listing of foods that contain trans fat:

- Most cookies
- Crackers
- Bake Mixes
- Donuts
- Stuffing Mixes
- Candy
- Bakery products
- Ice cream
- Drink Mixes
- Peanut Butter
- Bread
- Frozen food entrees
- Coffee creamers
- Breakfast cereals
- Breakfast bars
- Microwave popcorn
- Fried foods
- Cool whip

### Omega-6 Fats

Omega-6 fatty acids, also known as polyunsaturated fatty acids, are found in vegetable oils. They are essential for health when they are consumed in the right proportion to omega-3 fatty acids (discussed in the next section). They play a role in brain function, help stimulate the growth of the hair and skin, regulate metabolism, and help to maintain the reproductive system.

There are two problems with omega-6 fats. The first problem is the over-consumption of omega-6 fats as they relate to the consumption of omega 3 fats. Experts vary in their opinion on the ideal ratio of omega-3 fats to omega-6 fats. Some report that the ideal ratio for optimal brain functioning is 1:1: for every 1 gram of omega-6 fat, you need 1 gram of omega-3. Others report that a ratio of 3:1 is ideal for overall health: for every 3 grams of omega-6 fat, 1 gram of omega-3 fat should be consumed. However, health experts are agreement that most Americans have a ratio of 20 grams of omega-6 fat to 1 gram of omega-3 fat. This imbalance is believed to be a cause of inflammation in the body.

Secondly, most omega-6 fats that people consume are rancid. Rancid fat is a fat that has been exposed to too much light, heat, moisture and/or air, and has become rancid. The supermarket shelves are loaded with rancid fats. Most corn, soybean, canola, and peanut oil that is on the shelf in the supermarket in clear bottles is rancid because of the light it is exposed to in the supermarket. The only exception to this is olive oil, and it is preferable that you purchase olive oil in a dark glass container. Another good choice for fresh oil is flaxseed oil, which is located in the refrigerated section of the grocery store. It is best to buy small amounts of oil at a time to avoid rancidity.

Just about all commercially prepared salad dressings contain rancid oil as well. It is best that you make your own salad dressings from olive oil, adding in other ingredients to your liking. Also, omega-6 fats are found in processed foods. If you read a food label you will find overwhelmingly the fat of choice is an omega-6 fat such as soybean, corn, safflower, or sunflower. These processed omega-6 fats are a major source of the omega-6 fats that most people consume.

Your body needs omega-6 fats, but you want them from a healthy source. Below are  sources of unprocessed omega-6 fats:

- Flax seeds, flax seed oil, flax seed meal
- Hemp seeds, hemp seed oil
- Grapeseed Oil
- Pumpkin seeds, pumpkin seed oil
- Walnut oil
- Pine nuts
- Pistachio nuts
- Sesame Oil
- Sunflower seeds (raw)
- Olive oil, olives

## *Omega-3 Fats: The Good Guys*

Omega-3 fatty acids are also known as polyunsaturated fatty acids and are essential for good health. They are found in fish such as salmon, tuna, and halibut; other seafood, including algae and krill; chia seeds; some plants; walnuts, and nut oils. The American Heart Association recommends eating fish (particularly fatty fish such as mackerel, lake trout, herring, sardines, albacore tuna, and salmon) at least two times a week.

The University of Maryland Medical Center reports:

> *Research shows that omega-3 fatty acids reduce inflammation and may help lower the risk of chronic diseases such as heart disease, cancer, and arthritis. Omega-3 fatty acids are highly concentrated in the brain and appear to be important for cognitive (brain memory and performance) and behavioral function. In fact, infants who do not get enough omega-3 fatty acids from their mothers during pregnancy are at risk for developing vision and nerve problems. Symptoms of omega-3 fatty acid deficiency include fatigue, poor memory, dry skin, heart problems, mood swings or depression, and poor circulation.*

Restaurant meals are big on unhealthy fats. If you have ever watched some of the shows on The Food Network, especially *Diners, Drive-ins and Dives* with Guy Fiere, you know that fat appears to be the main ingredient in the food. The chart that follows  lists some meals at chain restaurants that are the worst offenders when it comes to fat content. Keep in mind that the average woman needs around 2,000 calories per day and 65 grams of fat, and the average man needs 2,500 calories per day with 65 grams of fat.

## Source: The Nation's Biggest Fat Bombs

http://blogs.indystar.com/fitforlife/2011/11/30/the-nations-biggest-fat-bombs-avoid-them/

| Restaurant | Menu Item | Calories | Fat Content |
|---|---|---|---|
| Ruby Tuesday | Triple Prime Bacon Cheddar Burger | 1,333 calories | 101 grams of fat |
| Chili's | Flame-Grilled Ribeye with broccoli and mashed potatoes | 1,460 calories | 106 grams of fat |

| International House of Pancakes | Chicken and Spinach Salad | 1,600 calories | 118 grams of fat |
|---|---|---|---|
| Applebee's | New England Fish and Chips | 1,930 calories | 138 grams of fat |
| Chili's | Bacon Ranch Chicken Quesadilla | 1,650 calories | 107 grams of fat |
| Cheesecake Factory | Fettuccini Alfredo with Chicken | 2300 calories | 103 grams of fat |

## POINT #3: WHY FRUITS AND VEGETABLES ARE SO IMPORTANT

Fruits and vegetables are the cornerstone of good health. The contain antioxidants and other phytonutrients that are complex and synergistic working in a magical way to support your health. While certain antioxidant vitamins have been reproduced in a laboratory and sold as a vitamin supplement, the thousands of phytonutrients have not been and the only source for them are fruits and vegetables. There are over 10,000 phytonutrients in one orange! Try making a vitamin with 10,000 ingredients and it would probably be as large as a pancake!

Think of your body as a machine. Like all machines, it needs fuel to make it run properly. The fuel that you provide your body is the food that you eat and the air that you breathe. As your body burns the fuel and reacts with the oxygen that you breathe, a process called oxidation is taking place inside of your cells. This process of oxidation produces free radicals.

Free radicals interact with other molecules within cells and can cause oxidative damage to the cells. Oxidative stress is a term used to define a condition in the body when the free radicals have gone amuck and are destroying your healthy cells. Free radical damage and oxidative stress lay the foundation for a host of diseases in your body.

There is only one way to keep free radicals from wreaking havoc in your body, and that is to make sure you have plenty of antioxidants in your body to arrest their activity, and the richest source of antioxidants are found in fruits and vegetables.

I have heard it said that not getting enough antioxidants in your diet is the same as irradiating yourself—you might as well stand in front of an X-ray machine unprotected! Consider the following statements:

- The rate of aging is nutrition and oxidative stress dependent (Dubois, 1998).
- Clearly free radical damage underlies much of aging which ultimately determines our health and our maximum life span....Free radical damage increases with age and is less well contained by and repaired by aged cells. (Weindruch & Rajindar, 1997).

The USDA recommends that all adults have a minimum of 4 servings of fruit and five servings of vegetables per day. A serving size is one-half of a cup. According to the study State of the Plate (2010) only 6% of individuals in the U.S. achieve this recommended target for vegetables and 8% achieve this recommended target for fruit in an average day.

Fruits and vegetables are the cornerstone of good nutrition and can protect you from a host of diseases. One-hundred-fifty scientists reviewed 4,500 research studies on the relationship between nutrition and cancer. They found overwhelming evidence that fruits, vegetables, and whole grains can prevent cancer. Their report states that 3 to 4 million cases of cancer could be prevented annually by modification in diet. (Dubois, 1998).

Many health professionals recommend taking the antioxidants as vitamin supplements, especially vitamins E, A, & C. While on the surface this may seem like a good idea, if you dig a little deeper, you will find some puzzling facts. There is no evidence that getting your antioxidants from a vitamin protects your health. Studies have shown quite the contrary.

- A study of 29,133 Finnish male smokers sought to determine if supplementation with vitamin A or vitamin E would prevent cancer and heart attacks in this group. The study was planned for ten years. After eight years it was stopped because:

  1. Supplementation with vitamin A showed an 18 percent increase in the incidence of lung cancer, and an 8 percent increase in overall mortality.
  2. Supplementation with vitamin E showed a 50 percent greater risk of hemorrhagic stroke and a 2 percent increase in overall mortality. (*New England Journal of Medicine,* 1994)

- The evidence is insufficient to recommend for or against the use of supplements of vitamins A, C, or E; multivitamins with folic acid; or antioxidant combinations for the prevention of cancer or cardiovascular disease (United States Preventive Task Force, 2003).

- Researchers from the University of Minnesota examined data from more than 38,000 women taking part in the Iowa Women's Health Study, an ongoing study with women who were around age sixty-two at its start in 1986. The researchers collected data on the women's supplement use in 1986, 1997, and 2004. Women who took supplements had, on average, a 2.4 percent increased risk of dying over the course of the nineteen-year study, compared with women who didn't take supplements, after the researchers adjusted for factors including the women's age and calorie intake. The study author states, *"Our study, as well as other similar studies, have provided very little evidence that commonly used dietary supplements would help to prevent chronic diseases."*(MSN.com)

While it is clear that a diet rich in fruits and vegetables is protective of your health, the jury is still out on vitamin supplements. The truth is that God knew what he was doing when he made a stalk of broccoli, a vine-ripened tomato, and oranges on a tree. The thousands of phytonutrients contained in fruits and vegetables work synergistically with one another in protecting you from sickness and disease, and this process cannot be duplicated by taking isolated vitamins and minerals.

If you cannot or will not eat the recommended four servings of fruit and five servings of vegetables per day, I recommend that you take a product called Juice Plus+®. I was introduced to this product over twelve years ago and immediately knew that I was on to something powerful. I have consumed it daily for the past twelve years and I know it will always be a part of my diet. It is my nutritional safety net for those days when I do not have access to the types and amounts of fruits and vegetables that my body needs.

*Juice Plus+*® contains seventeen different fruits and vegetables that have been juiced, with the water, sugar, and salt removed. It is then dried at a cool temperature, and the resultant powder is placed in gelatin capsules. I find it to be the next best thing to fruits and vegetables. I know exactly what is in it because they did not stray too far from God's original design. I can also trust *Juice Plus+*® because of the dozens of excellent research projects that have been completed on *Juice Plus+*® with impressive results. Per their official website, some of the research shows:

- *Juice Plus+*® *delivers key phytonutrients that are absorbed by the body.*
- *Juice Plus+*® *reduces oxidative stress.*
- *Juice Plus+*® *positively impacts markers of systemic inflammation.*
- *Juice Plus+*® *helps support a healthy immune system.*
- *Juice Plus+*® *helps protect DNA.*
- *Juice Plus+*® *positively impacts several key indicators of cardiovascular wellness.*

In the spirit of full disclosure, I am a licensed distributor for *Juice Plus+*®. The product can be ordered at www.realhealthfood.com. If you choose to purchase *Juice Plus+*® at this website, the author will receive a financial remuneration from your purchase.

## POINT #4: THE WHITER THE BREAD, THE QUICKER YOU'RE DEAD!

White flour is a devitalized foodstuff that is destroying the health of anyone who consumes it on a regular basis. It may be pleasing to an adulterated palate that can no longer appreciate the rich-bodied taste of whole grains, but it wreaks havoc in the body. Every time I think about how white flour products have so permeated our culture, this scripture comes to mind:

> *Why do you spend money for what is not bread, And your wages for what does not satisfy? Listen carefully to Me, and eat what is good, And let your soul delight itself in abundance. Isaiah 55:2 (NKJV)*

White bread is not bread; it is white fluff stuff! It does not satisfy your body's nutritional needs and consuming it does not bring about abundant health. One of my favorite laments is that I work too hard for my money to give it away to merchants who are out to destroy my health! A chant that I have my audience sing in my workshops is:

> "Making you rich, but making me sick."

Like it or not, this is the truth about how many people spend their food dollars.

## WHOLE WHEAT FLOUR VS. WHITE FLOUR

| Whole Wheat Flour | White Flour |
| --- | --- |
| Whole wheat flour is made from the entire wheat grain:<br><br>The bran: This is the outer layer of the wheat grain and contains fiber<br><br>The endosperm: This is the middle layer, is the largest part of the wheat grain, and is mostly starch.<br><br>The germ: This is the innermost layer where the vitamins and nutrients are contained and what can be used to grow new wheat grains. | White flour is made from the endosperm, which is the starchiest part of flour. |
| 3 grams of fiber per serving | 1 gram of fiber per serving |
| 4 grams of protein per serving | 3 grams of protein per serving |
| 1 gram of fat per serving | 0 grams of fat per serving |
| Naturally occurring nutrients and vitamins in balance the way God intended | Artificially fortified with vitamins and minerals |
| -58 inflammation rating per serving | -101 inflammation rating per serving |

Have you ever wondered who came up with the idea of stripping whole-wheat flour of its natural ingredients to come up with white flour? From what I can glean, white flour came about because of the need (not really the need, but the opportunity) to mass-produce flour. With large quantities of flour being produced at once, concerns arose regarding the shelf life of the flour. The natural fatty acids, vitamins, and minerals in whole-wheat flour causes flour to become rancid after about 8 months or so. So the solution was to take away the part of the wheat, the germ, that contained vitamins and minerals, and the flour would have a longer shelf life. Now isn't that just what we needed—a food product so dead that bacteria bugs don't even want it!

White flour can be purchased bleached or unbleached. Ponder that one for a moment. Why are they bleaching food? I understand using bleach for whitening my laundry, but for flour? Really? The bleaching process involves the use of chemicals. There is debate as to the dangers of the chemicals used.

Danielle Kosecki, writing for *Prevention Magazine*, is of the opinion that the chemicals used in the bleaching of flour are safe. She states:

> *...Flour bleaches naturally on its own as yellow compounds called xanto-phylls react with oxygen in the air; this takes several weeks. To speed the whitening, processors bleach flour—turning it white from its natural straw color—with safe, FDA-regulated chemicals (some of the same ones used to sanitize veggies). Alloxan may form as a byproduct, but the amount is minuscule (less than 0.03 mg per slice of bread) and harmless...*

Joseph Mercola, a strong proponent of a no-grain diet and a natural health enthusiast, takes issue with the above statement. He argues:

> *...The milling industry now uses a gas known as chlorine oxide as an aging, bleaching, and oxidizing agent. Industry leaders claim that bleaching and oxidizing agents don't produce harmful residues in flour, but they can't cite published data or studies to confirm this. The Environmental Protection Agency warns that chlorine oxide is a dangerous irritant. Chlorine oxide interacts with some of the proteins in the flour and produces alloxan, a product of the decomposition of uric acid. Alloxan is a poison used to produce diabetes in healthy laboratory animals so that researchers can study diabetes "treatments..."*

Besides the fact that white flour has been stripped of its naturally occurring vitamins and minerals, it also lacks the fiber that is essential to bowel health. An adult needs a minimum of 25 grams of fiber per day in the diet, and two slices of whole wheat bread provide from between 6 to 8 grams of fiber. Bowel health is certainly not a topic you want to discuss at your next party, but from my conversations with people, most people are walking around constipated every day. Everyone should have a bowel movement at least two to three times a day. And the moving of the bowels should not require long bouts on the commode that require reading material. The moving of bowels should be just as quick as passing urine. If you are straining and grunting to move your bowels, you need added fiber in your diet, and the best source is the fiber contained in whole foods.

Many health experts believe that white flour may be partly the blame for the rise in type II diabetes. Without the bran and the germ in the flour, white flour quickly converts to sugar in your system. The challenges with too much sugar in your system are discussed later in the next section.

I recommend that if you are going to consume products made with wheat flour that you buy products made from 100 percent stone ground whole-wheat flour. This is different from a product that says "wheat flour." Wheat flour is white flour that has not been bleached, not whole grain wheat flour. If the first ingredient on the food label says wheat flour, the food is predominately white flour. Foods made with white flour include:

- Cookies
- Crackers
- Waffles
- Pancake mixes
- Donuts
- Pastries
- Tortillas
- Pretzels
- Pizza
- Bagels
- Breakfast cereals
- Wheat bread

White rice goes through a similar process of stripping just as wheat flour does. Brown rice is more nutritious and contains essential fiber and other nutrients for the maintenance of a healthy body.

## POINT #5: SUGAR BLUES

Our society is in love with sugar! Think about the cute names we give each other when we are in love: sugar, honey, sweetie pie, and cupcake. And ladies, what is it with the candy bars that are named after men: Mr. Goodbar, Oh, Henry! Sugar Daddy, 3 Musketeers.

According to Dr. Oz, the average person consumes 150 pounds of sugar per year—compared to just 7 ½ pounds consumed on average in the year 1700, which is 20 times as much!

White table sugar is refined and processed and contains no vitamins, no minerals, no enzymes, no fiber, and no nutritional value. Talk about empty calories! Sugar is a dead food and it only contributes to death in your body. One of my favorite things I like to do when I am doing a nutrition seminar is to show the audience a 5 pound bag of sugar from one of the major food companies, and ask someone to read the label on the side of the bag, which states:

QUALITY MAINTAINED INDEFINITELY IF STORED IN A COOL, DRY PLACE.

Does this sound like food to you? What food product do you know that can be maintained indefinitely?

According to Dr. Nancy Appleton, author of the book *Lick the Sugar Habit,* there are 76 ways in which sugar is bad for your health. I have bolded some of them to make sure you pay attention to it.

1. **Sugar can suppress your immune system and impair your defenses against infectious disease.**
2. Sugar upsets the mineral relationships in your body: causes chromium and copper deficiencies and interferes with absorption of calcium and magnesium.
3. Sugar can cause can cause a rapid rise of adrenaline, hyperactivity, anxiety, difficulty concentrating, and crankiness in children.
4. **Sugar can produce a significant rise in total cholesterol, triglycerides and bad cholesterol and a decrease in good cholesterol.**
5. Sugar causes a loss of tissue elasticity and function.
6. **Sugar feeds cancer cells and has been connected with the development of cancer of the breast, ovaries, prostate, rectum, pancreas, biliary tract, lung, gallbladder, and stomach.**
7. Sugar can increase fasting levels of glucose and can cause reactive hypoglycemia.
8. Sugar can weaken eyesight.
9. Sugar can cause many problems with the gastrointestinal tract, including an acidic digestive tract, indigestion, malabsorption in patients with functional bowel disease, increased risk of Crohn's disease, and ulcerative colitis.
10. **Sugar can cause premature aging.**
11. Sugar can lead to alcoholism.

12. Sugar can cause your saliva to become acidic, [leading to] tooth decay, and periodontal disease.
13. Sugar contributes to obesity.
14. **Sugar can cause autoimmune diseases such as arthritis, asthma, multiple sclerosis.**
15. Sugar greatly assists the uncontrolled growth of Candida Albicans (yeast infections).
16. Sugar can cause gallstones.
17. Sugar can cause appendicitis.
18. Sugar can cause hemorrhoids.
19. Sugar can cause varicose veins.
20. Sugar can elevate glucose and insulin responses in oral contraceptive users.
21. **Sugar can contribute to osteoporosis.**
22. Sugar can cause a decrease in your insulin sensitivity, thereby causing abnormally high insulin levels and eventually diabetes.
23. Sugar can lower your Vitamin E levels.
24. Sugar can increase your systolic blood pressure.
25. Sugar can cause drowsiness and decreased activity in children.
26. High sugar intake increases advanced glycation end products (AGEs) (Sugar molecules attaching to and thereby damaging proteins in the body).
27. Sugar can interfere with your absorption of protein.
28. Sugar causes food allergies.
29. Sugar can cause toxemia during pregnancy.
30. Sugar can contribute to eczema in children.
31. **Sugar can cause atherosclerosis and cardiovascular disease.**
32. Sugar can impair the structure of your DNA.
33. Sugar can change the structure of protein and cause a permanent alteration of the way the proteins act in your body.
34. Sugar can make your skin age by changing the structure of collagen.
35. Sugar can cause cataracts and nearsightedness.
36. Sugar can cause emphysema.

37.  High sugar intake can impair the physiological homeostasis of many systems in your body.

38.  Sugar lowers the ability of enzymes to function.

39.  **Sugar intake is higher in people with Parkinson's disease.**

40.  Sugar can increase the size of your liver by making your liver cells divide, and it can increase the amount of liver fat.

41.  Sugar can increase kidney size and produce pathological changes in the kidney such as the formation of kidney stones.

42.  Sugar can damage your pancreas.

43.  **Sugar can increase your body's fluid retention.**

44.  Sugar is enemy #1 of your bowel movement.

45.  Sugar can compromise the lining of your capillaries.

46.  Sugar can make your tendons more brittle.

47.  Sugar can cause headaches, including migraines.

48.  **Sugar can reduce the learning capacity, adversely affect school children's grades, and cause learning disorders.**

49.  Sugar can cause an increase in delta, alpha, and theta brain waves, which can alter your mind's ability to think clearly.

50.  **Sugar can cause depression.**

51.  Sugar can increase your risk of gout.

52.  **Sugar can increase your risk of Alzheimer's disease.**

53.  Sugar can cause hormonal imbalances such as increasing estrogen in men, exacerbating PMS, and decreasing growth hormone.

54.  Sugar can lead to dizziness.

55.  **Diets high in sugar will increase free radicals and oxidative stress.**

56.  High sucrose diets of subjects with peripheral vascular disease significantly increase platelet adhesion.

57.  High sugar consumption of pregnant adolescents can lead to substantial decrease in gestation duration and is associated with a twofold increased risk for delivering a small-for-gestational-age (SGA) infant.

58.  **Sugar is an addictive substance.**

59.  Sugar can be intoxicating, similar to alcohol.

60.   Sugar given to premature babies can affect the amount of carbon dioxide they produce.

61.   Decrease in sugar intake can increase emotional stability.

62.   **Your body changes sugar into two to five times more fat in the bloodstream than it does starch.**

63.   The rapid absorption of sugar promotes excessive food intake in obese subjects.

64.   Sugar can worsen the symptoms of children with attention deficit hyperactivity disorder (ADHD).

65.   Sugar adversely affects urinary electrolyte composition.

66.   Sugar can slow down the ability of your adrenal glands to function.

67.   Sugar has the potential of inducing abnormal metabolic processes in a normal healthy individual and promoting chronic degenerative diseases.

68.   I.V.s (intravenous feedings) of sugar water can cut off oxygen to your brain.

69.   Sugar increases your risk of polio.

70.   High sugar intake can cause epileptic seizures.

71.   Sugar causes high blood pressure in obese people.

72.   In intensive care units, limiting sugar saves lives.

73.   Sugar may induce cell death.

74.   In juvenile rehabilitation camps, when children were put on a low sugar diet, there was a 44 percent drop in antisocial behavior.

75.   Sugar dehydrates newborns.

76.   Sugar can cause gum disease.

Do you need any more reasons to limit sugar in your diet? I think not. I urge you to begin today reducing/eliminating sugar from your daily diet.

### High Fructose Corn Syrup (HFCS)

HFCS is a common sweetener and preservative that is made by changing the glucose in cornstarch to fructose, which is another form of sugar. The end product is a combination of fructose and glucose  It was introduced into the U.S. food supply in 1967, and now accounts for 40 percent of the sugars ingested in the U.S. (Bray, Nielsen, & Popkin, 2004).

The rise in obesity in the U.S. also correlates with the rise in the use of HFCS in the food supply (Bray, et al, 2004). Bray and his team of researchers, based on analysis of what occurs when an individual consumes HFCS versus table sugar, are of the opinion that consumption of HFCS is at least partially the blame for the obesity epidemic. They explain that HFCS has a different metabolic effect on the system than other sugars.

When the sugar glucose (table sugar) enters your bloodstream, your body releases the hormone insulin to help regulate it. Fructose does not enter your bloodstream the way glucose does because fructose is processed in your liver. When you consume a lot of fructose at one time, such as when you are drinking a soda that has been sweetened with HFCS, the liver cannot process it fast enough for your body to use it as sugar. So your liver begins to churn out fats from the fructose in the form of triglycerides, and these triglycerides are what enter your bloodstream. As noted earlier in our discussion of triglycerides, they are a type of fat found in your blood, which may contribute to hardening of the arteries. Hardening of the arteries increases the risk of stroke, diabetes, heart attack and heart disease.

Another concern is that when you consume glucose, your body releases the hormone insulin to regulate it, but it also releases the hormone leptin. Leptin helps to regulate food intake and helps you know you are full. Fructose does not trigger the release of leptin as fructose is processed in your liver. Without this inhibitory effect of leptin, your body's normal appetite suppressant system is overridden. Hence, individuals are prone to eat more.

My advice is to totally eliminate HFCS from your diet. Like partially hydrogenated oil, it is ubiquitous and is in most processed food.

### *Recommended Daily Amount of Sugar*

Recommendations from the American Heart Association — not a part of official U.S. dietary guidelines — say that most American women should consume no more than 100 calories (six teaspoons) a day from added sugar from any source, and that most American men should consume no more than 150 calories (nine teaspoons) a day from added sugar, and that even less is better. Added sugar does not include the sugar you find naturally in fruit, vegetables, and dairy products.

You can easily get six to nine teaspoons of added sugar in your diet without ever lifting a spoon of sugar. Sugar is disguised by other names. Although some of these other sugars are natural and may have a few trace minerals, they are all still sugar. They are listed alphabetically below.

- Agave nectar
- Barley malt syrup
- Brown sugar
- Corn sweetener
- Corn syrup, or corn syrup solids
- Dehydrated cane juice
- Dextrin
- Dextrose
- Fructose
- Fruit juice concentrate
- Glucose
- High-fructose corn syrup
- Honey
- Invert sugar
- Lactose
- Maltodextrin
- Malt syrup
- Maltose
- Maple syrup
- Molasses
- Raw sugar
- Rice syrup
- Saccharose
- Sorghum or sorghum syrup
- Sucrose
- Sucanat
- Syrup
- Treacle
- Turbinado sugar
- Xylosehoney

*Artificial Sweeteners*

Many individuals use artificial sweeteners so they can still enjoy the taste of sweet food without adding extra calories. The artificial sweeteners currently approved by the Food and Drug Administration (FDA) are:

- Acesulfame potassium (Sunett, Sweet One)
- Aspartame (Equal, NutraSweet)
- Neotame
- Saccharin (SugarTwin, Sweet'N Low)
- Sucralose (Splenda)

The FDA has determined that these substances are safe and can be included as a regular part of your diet without any deleterious health effects.

Many holistic health practitioners, including this author, disagree. Artificial sweeteners are just that: artificial. They are not real food. They are the product of chemicals and substances that have been manipulated in a laboratory. One rule I would like to encourage you to use when you are deciding whether a food is safe for your body is to ask yourself:

- Can I trace this back to what God made for me to eat?
- If I can trace it back to a natural food, how many steps away is this from what God intended?
- Is this a fake food or a real food?

Eating natural foods will not only improve your health, but it will improve your weight as well.

Several studies have raised concern regarding the safety of artificial sweeteners. As reported by medical author Melissa Conrad Stöppler in the article "Aspartame Safety Concerns":

*In response to research published by Italian scientists that suggests that the artificial sweetener aspartame can cause cancer, the U.S. consumer organization Center for Science in the Public Interest requested an urgent Food and Drug Administration (FDA) review of the product's safety in June 2007.*

*…The data that sparked the controversy were from a report by researchers at the European Ramazzini Foundation (ERF) in Bologna, Italy, published in 2005. The scientists carried out tests of over 4,000 rats that regularly*

*consumed high doses of aspartame and were allowed to live until they died naturally. Scientists from ERF concluded from their study that aspartame causes cancer and that current uses and consumption of the sweetener should be reevaluated…*

*…The European Food Safety Authority (EFSA)… and the FDA evaluated the data from the study and concluded that they would support their currently held positions that aspartame was safe.*

Another concern with artificial sweeteners is that they continue to stimulate your appetite for sweet foods. Also, because so-called diet foods contain artificial sweeteners and fewer calories, many people are eating more of the so-called diet food because it is lower in calories, and they end up eating more than if they had eaten something sweetened with natural sugar.

## Stevia

Stevia is not an artificial sweetener but is a natural non-caloric herb that has been used for thousands of years in many parts of the world. Its plant name is rebiana, and it is grown in many parts of South America and other tropical and sub-tropical regions. It has a sweetness of about 200 to 300 times that of sugar, depending on the form that you purchase it in. It can be purchased in liquid or powder form.

It is marketed in most supermarkets under the name Truvia and PureVia in powder form. Both Truvia and PureVia mix in a sweetener called Erythritol. Erythritol is a substitute low-calorie sugar-alcohol (see below). In addition to both products adding erythritol, PureVia adds a sweetener called isomaltulose.

I've yet to see any negative reports or health concerns regarding the use of stevia. I use it in small amounts occasionally and prefer the powder form. My hesitancy with stevia is the level of laboratory processes that it undergoes before it gets to market. I am of the opinion that once a large manufacturer starts to produce anything in mass quantities, something is bound to go awry.

## Sugar Alcohols

Sugar alcohols are reduced-calorie sweeteners. The name is very misleading because they contain neither sugar or alcohol. They are made by adding hydrogen to sugar molecules so the body ignores them. On average, sugar alcohols provide about half the calories of sugar and other carbohydrates, and they are often used by diabetics. They have been known to have a laxative effect and can cause gastrointestinal distress.

While sugar alcohols have been determined by the FDA to be safe, my same rule applies: Is this what God did? Do you really want something in your body that has been chemically altered?

The American Diabetic Association (www.diabetes.org) offers this advice for calculating the net effect of sugar alcohol in your diet:

If a food has more than 5 grams of sugar alcohols:
- Subtract ½ the grams of sugar alcohol from the amount of total carbohydrate
- Count the remaining grams of carbohydrate in your meal plan
- Example:
  o Portion: 1 bar
  o Total carbohydrate 15 grams, total sugar alcohol 6 grams.
  o One half of 6 is 3, 15 minus 3 = 12.
  o Hence, one bar counts as 12 grams carbohydrate

Examples of sugar alcohols are:
- erythritol
- hydrogenated starch hydrolysates
- isomalt
- lactitol
- maltitol
- mannitol
- sorbitol
- xylitol

## POINT # 6: SALT

A diet high in salt is not good for your health. Too much salt in the diet can lead to hypertension, which can lead to stroke and heart attack. High salt diets have been linked to increased inflammation in the body. High salt diets lead to the body retaining fluids, making you look and feel bloated. High salt diets may also be linked to increased risk for osteoporosis. Sellmeyer, Schloetter, and Sebastian (2002) note that:

*The impact of abundant dietary salt on skeletal health has yet to be established, but {it} is potentially detrimental through increased urinary calcium losses.*

The 2010 Dietary Guidelines for Americans recommend limiting sodium to less than 2,300 mg a day. The recommendation drops to 1,500 mg per day if you're age fifty-one or older, are African American, have high blood pressure, diabetes, or chronic kidney disease. The average American consumes 2–3 times the recommended amount. Most of the salt a person consumes does not come from the salt shaker on the table, but from the excessive amounts of salt that is in processed foods. Canned soups are notorious for their salt content, as well as pre-packaged frozen foods and restaurant foods.

Below are examples of salt gone amuck at some of America's favorite restaurants. Remember that the recommended daily allowance (RDA) of fat is 65 grams.

## SOURCE: EAT THIS, NOT THAT

http://eatthis.menshealth.com/content/6-saltiest-comfort-food

| Restaurant | Dish | Nutritional Analysis | Salt Equivalent |
|---|---|---|---|
| Denny's | Meat Loaf Dinner (with mashed potatoes and corn) | Sodium 5,080 mg Calories 1,210 Fat 69 g | 100 cups of popcorn |
| Papa John's | Cheese sticks with Buffalo Sauce | Sodium 6,700 mg Calories 2,605 Fat 113 g | 20 orders of McDonald's large French fries |
| Pizza Hut Meat | Meat Lover's Stuffed Crust Pizza (3 slices of the 14" large) | Sodium 5,070 mg Calories 1,560 Fat 87 g | 34 strips of bacon |
| Chili's | Buffalo Chicken Fajitas | Sodium 5,690 Calories 1,750 Fat 107 | 3½ pounds of salted peanuts |

| P.F. Chang's | Beef with Broccoli | Sodium 3,752 mg<br>Calories 1,120<br>Fat 65 g | 6 large orders of Burger King onion rings |
| Romano's | Macaroni Grill Chicken Portobello | Sodium 7,300 mg<br>Calories: 1,020<br>Fat 66 g | 48 strips of bacon |

## POINT #7: WATER VS. SWEETENED BEVERAGES

Water is the health elixir for all ages. You simply cannot improve on God's design to quench your thirst and cleanse your body. Zero calories and in abundant supply, water is one of the best tools to include in your healthy living arsenal.

Your body is mostly made of water—a whopping 66 percent! This figure varies per medical source, and I have seen a figure quoted up to 73 percent. Your brain is about 70 percent water, your blood 80 percent, skin 44 percent, muscles 75 percent, and bone 22 percent.

Water is essential for life. You can go for days, weeks, and even a month without solid food, but without water your life would end in about a week or less. Next to oxygen, water is the most important thing that you need to sustain your life.

Listed below are the important roles that water plays in your body.

- Water helps to regulate your body temperature.
- Water removes waste and toxins from your body.
- Water keeps your joints lubricated.
- Water transports vital nutrients to your organs.
- Water can help maintain a healthy body weight.
- Water helps to suppress your appetite.
- The most common cause of fatigue is dehydration.
- In some people the thirst mechanism is so weak that they think they are hungry when they really are thirsty.
- By the time you feel thirsty your body is already mildly dehydrated.
- Drinking adequate amounts of water reduces your risk for certain cancers including colon, bladder, and breast cancer.
- Water improves the appearance of your skin.

- Water combats constipation.
- Waters helps with the digestion of your food.

For the most part, I only drink water and unsweetened green or herbal tea. It has been over a dozen years since I drank a soda. I avoid all sweetened drinks like the plague, and if I have to succumb to one, that is usually because there is no other source of water available other than a public drinking fountain or water from a public bathroom faucet—and I always pass on both. In restaurants when my fellow diners are ordering coffee, I often order a cup of hot water. This always throws the waiter off and they ask me if I want tea. I respond, no I just want a cup of hot water. They will go on to ask if I want lemon with it, and I just politely smile and respond, "A *cup of plain hot water is fine.*" What usually follows is a puzzled but resigned expression on the waiter's face. I guess I am the only one that drinks hot water.

How much water should you drink per day? The number of ounces varies according to whom you are talking to. The standard answer is 64 ounces, which is eight, eight-ounce glasses. This really isn't that hard to do, since most households use 12- or 16-ounce glasses. My trick for making sure I drink at least 64 ounces of water a day is to drink 16 ounces of warm water as soon as I wake up. Supposedly, this does all kinds of great things for detoxifying my liver—I just know that it helps me to get one-fourth of my daily requirement of water out of the way!

### Fruit Juice

Fruit juices have been touted as being healthy for you. They are indeed a healthy alternative to soda, but there is a dark side to fruit juice. Without the added fiber that is contained in the whole piece of fruit, the sugar from the juice rushes into your bloodstream unimpeded by fiber. This causes a surge of insulin into your body, as compared to what would happen if the sugar from fruit were introduced more slowly as when you eat a whole piece of fruit.

Research has shown that a glass of fruit juice can contain more calories than a glass of soda. Most fruit juices are very high in fructose, a simple sugar commonly associated with obesity due to its quick conversion to fat. Even though the fructose in fruit juice is natural compared to the toxic high fructose corn syrup most often used to sweeten soda, natural fructose still goes straight to the liver where it quickly metabolizes.

Many commercial juices are pasteurized and processed, and by the time they end up in your glass, many of the important nutrients have been lost. Would it surprise you to learn that orange juice labeled "fresh squeezed, not from concentrate" has been languishing in a storage vat for up to one year? It's best to freshly squeeze or juice your fruit if you want fruit juice.

A piece of whole fruit is rich in fiber, antioxidants, and other vital nutrients that work in conjunction with one another to nourish the body. Most fruit juice has been stripped of all these things during processing, rendering a juice that is high in sugar but low in nutrients. A glass of commercial apple juice, for instance, has six apples' worth of fructose and none of the fiber and pulp that helps to properly assimilate that sugar into the body. The result is an overload of sugar that floods the liver, increasing the risk of diabetes and heart disease.

## Soda

You are already aware that the sugar in soda is bad for your health and contributes to weight gain. Not only does soda contribute to weight gain, but a new study found that drinking two or more sugary beverages per day increases a woman's risk for heart disease and diabetes even if it does not make her gain weight. The women in the study who drank two or more sugary beverages also had higher amounts of belly fat, which poses a greater cardiovascular risk than other types of fat.

The phosphoric acid in colas depletes the body of magnesium, which the brain uses for many functions and  is vital to the body's production of energy. Consuming one can of soda with phosphoric acid can cause you to lose 36 mg of magnesium (Klapp, 2011).

The Academy of General Dentistry (AGD) journal *General Dentistry*, reports that drinking any type of soft drink hurts teeth due to the citric acid and/or phosphoric acid in the beverages (Lloyd, 2007).

Studies have linked consumption of sodas to increased risk for osteoporosis. Researchers at Tufts University in Boston reported that among the 1,413 women whose dietary records and bone-density scans they reviewed, those who drank a diet or regular cola at least three times a week over five years had significantly lower bone densities than those who sipped cola once a month or less (Hendley, 2008).

## Diet Soda

Linda Carroll, a reporter for msnbc.com, reported on a study which followed more than 2,500 New Yorkers for nine or more years and found that people who drank diet soda every day had a 61 percent higher risk of vascular events, including stroke and heart attack, than those who completely eschewed the diet drinks. The increased likelihood of vascular events remained even after the study authors accounted for risk factors, such as smoking, high blood pressure, and high cholesterol levels. The researchers found no increased risk among people who drank regular soda.

Carroll further reported that a physician at a leading hospital in Pennsylvania noted that this was the second study to associate diet soda with health issues. An earlier study found that diet soda consumption was linked to an increased risk of metabolic syndrome. Metabolic syndrome is a cluster of conditions — increased blood pressure, a high blood sugar level, excess body fat around the waist or abnormal cholesterol levels — that occur together, increasing your risk of heart disease, stroke and diabetes (Mayo Clinic).

Carroll states that the physician also reported that there are animal studies suggesting a link between vascular problems and caramel-containing products. Caramel is the ingredient that gives the dark color to sodas like Coke and Pepsi.

In June 2011, Leah Goldman reported that data from a recent study by the American Diabetes Association showed that while diet sodas may be free of calories, they do not prevent you from gaining weight. In fact, they may contribute to weight gain. The ADA analyzed measures of height, weight, and waist circumference compared to diet soda consumption over a period of nine-and-a-half years and found that the adults who drank more diet soda per day gained more weight and added to their waistlines. Diet soda also contributes to diabetes, heart disease, cancer, and other chronic conditions.

Dr. Mike Dow, a contributing physician on the website Sharecare, which is in partnership with Johns Hopkins Medicine (www.sharecare.com) states:

*One study showed 41 percent increase in risk of being overweight for every can of diet soda consumed every day! You can recalibrate your taste buds, so even if the diet soda has no calories, the hundreds-of-times-sweeter-than-sugar taste takes away your ability to appreciate the more subtle sweetness of things like whole fruit. And you may then need very sweet foods to get the same perception of sweetness.*

Dr. Michael Roizen, also a contributing physician on Sharecare writes:

*Even drinking diet drinks is associated with a higher risk of metabolic syndrome. Consumption of sugar (or its equivalents, like corn syrup) in soft drinks has been linked to obesity in children and adolescents. But a recent study of almost all 50-year-old men and women in Framingham, Massachusetts, found that having more than one soft drink daily, whether sugared or diet, increased the risk of metabolic syndrome by 44 percent over a four-year period. The risk was increased similarly whether the drink was sugared or diet.*

One theory is that the high sweetness of drinks conditions people to crave sweet foods; another is that ingredients in the drinks can lead to insulin resistance or inflammation.

I trust that all of the above facts about sweetened beverages have convinced you to make water your beverage of choice. Listed below are some other facts about water that you may find interesting.

- Roughly 70 percent of an adult's body is made up of water.
- At birth, water accounts for approximately 80 percent of an infant's body weight.
- A healthy person can drink about three gallons (48 cups) of water per day.
- Drinking too much water too quickly can lead to water intoxication. Water intoxication occurs when water dilutes the sodium level in the bloodstream and causes an imbalance of water in the brain.
- Water intoxication is most likely to occur during periods of intense athletic performance.
- While the daily recommended amount of water is eight cups per day, not all of this water must be consumed in the liquid form. Nearly every food or drink item provides some water to the body.

- Soft drinks, coffee, and tea, while made up almost entirely of water, also contain caffeine. Caffeine can act as a mild diuretic, preventing water from traveling to necessary locations in the body.
- Pure water (solely hydrogen and oxygen atoms) has a neutral pH of 7, which is neither acidic nor basic.
- Water dissolves more substances than any other liquid. Wherever it travels, water carries chemicals, minerals, and nutrients with it.
- Somewhere between 70 and 75 percent of the earth's surface is covered with water.
- Much more fresh water is stored under the ground in aquifers than on the earth's surface.
- The earth is a closed system, similar to a terrarium, meaning that it rarely loses or gains extra matter. The same water that existed on the earth millions of years ago is still present today.
- The total amount of water on the earth is about 326 million cubic miles of water.
- Of all the water on the earth, humans can use only about three tenths of a percent of this water. Such usable water is found in groundwater aquifers, rivers, and freshwater lakes.
- The United States uses nearly 80 percent of its water for irrigation and thermoelectric power.
- The average person in the United States uses anywhere from 80–100 gallons of water per day. Flushing the toilet actually takes up the largest amount of this water.
- Approximately 85 percent of U.S. residents receive their water from public water facilities. The remaining 15 percent supply their own water from private wells or other sources.
- By the time a person feels thirsty, his or her body has lost over 1 percent of its total water amount.
- The weight a person loses directly after intense physical activity is weight from water, not fat.

## REFERENCES FOR CHAPTER THREE

American Heart Association. *A history of trans fat.* Accessed November 10, 2011 at http://www.heart.org/HEARTORG/GettingHealthy/FatsAndOils/Fats101/A-History-of-Trans-Fat_UCM_301463_Article.jsp

Applegate, N. *Lick the sugar habit.* Accessed November 20, 2011 at http://articles.mercola.com/sites/articles/archive/2005/05/04/sugar-dangers-part-two.aspxasis.

Bray, G.A., Nielsen, S.J., & Popkin, B.M. (2004). *Consumption of high-fructose corn syrup in beverages may play a role in the obesity epidemic* [Electronic version]. *The American Journal of Clinical Nutrition,* 79(4), 537-543.

Carper, J. (2000) *Your miracle brain.* New York: HarperCollins.

Carroll, L. (2011) *Daily diet soda tied to higher risk for stroke, heart attack.* Accessed September 20, 2011 at http://www.msnbc.msn.com/id/41479869/ns/health-diet_and_nutrition/t/daily-diet-soda-tied-higher-risk-stroke-heart-attack

Dubois, R. (1998). *Oxidative stress in the pathogenesis of disease and aging: Opportunity for intervention.*

Franklin Institute Resources for Science Learning. *The human brain.* Accessed September 3, 2011 at http://www.fi.edu/learn/brain/fats.html

Goldman, L. (2011). *Bad news, Your "diet" soda is making you fat too.* http://articles.businessinsider.com/2011-06-29/news/30010277_1_diet-soda-weight-gain-aspartame

Hendley, J. (2008). *Can Drinking Seltzers, Sodas, or Other Carbonated Drinks Harm Bones?* Accessed September 20, 2011 at http://www.eatingwell.com/nutrition_health/bone_health/can_drinking_seltzers_sodas_or_other_carbonated_drinks_harm_bones

Klapp, E. (2011). Accessed September 29, 2011 at http://www.sharecare.com/question/why-soda-bad-for-health

Kosecki, D. *Is white flour bleached with dangerous chemicals?* Prevention Magazine. Accessed January 12, 2012 at http://www.prevention.com/white-flour-health-risks

Lloyd, R. (2007). *Acids in popular sodas erode tooth enamel.* Accessed September 29, 2011 at http://www.livescience.com/7198-acids-popular-sodas-erode-tooth-enamel.html

Mayo Clinic. *Metabolic Syndrome.* Accessed March 15, 2012 at http://www.mayoclinic.com/health/metabolic%20syndrome/DS00522

Mercola, J. *The little known secrets about bleached flour.* Accessed January 12, 2012 at http://articles.mercola.com/sites/articles/archive/2009/03/26/The-Little-Known-Secrets-about-Bleached-Flour.aspx

MSN.com. *Too much vitamins dangerous for women: Study.* Accessed October 20, 2011 at http://news.in.msn.com/international/article.aspx?cp-documentid=5504685

Omega 3 fatty acids. University of Maryland Medical Center. Accessed September 12, 2011 at http://www.umm.edu/altmed/articles/omega-3-000316.htm

Oz, M. Answers the question how much sugar do Americans consume annually. Accessed January 20, 2012 at http://www.sharecare.com/question/sugar-consume-every-year).

Sellmeyer, D.E., Schloetter, M., and Sebastian A. (2002) *Potassium citrate prevents increased urine calcium excretion and bone resorption induced by a high sodium chloride diet.* [Electronic version]. Journal of Clinical Endocrinology Metabolism. Vol 87, pp. 2008-12.

State of the Plate: 2010 Study on America's Consumption of Fruits and Vegetables (2010).  Produce for Better Health Foundation.  Accessed February 5, 2012 at http://www.pbhfoundation.org.

Stöppler, M. C. (2007). *Aspartame Safety Concerns.* Accessed September 18, 2011 at http://www.medicinenet.com/script/main/art.asp?articlekey=82425

The New England Journal of Medicine (1994). *The effect of vitamin E and beta carotene on the incidence of lung cancer and other cancers in male smokers.* [Electronic version] Vol. 330:1029-1035

*Twenty Interesting and Useful Water Facts.* Accessed March 10, 2012 at http://www.allaboutwater.org/water-facts.html

United States Preventive Task Force (2003) *Routine vitamin supplementation to prevent cancer and cardiovascular disease.* Routine Annals of Internal Medicine: Vol. 139, pp. 56-70)

University of Maryland Medical Center. *Omega-3 fatty acids.* Accessed January 15, 2012 at http://www.umm.edu/altmed/articles/omega-3-000316.htm

Weil, A. *Rethinking saturated fat.* Accessed January 24, 2012 at http://www.drweil.com/drw/u/QAA400919/Rethinking-Saturated-Fat.html

Weindruch, R. & Sohal R. (1997) *Calorie intake and aging.* New England Journal of Medicine [Electronic version]. Vol. 33, pp. 986-994.

# CHAPTER FOUR
## EXERCISE

Do you know what the best exercise in the world is? Did you guess walking, swimming, biking, hiking, or running? Nope. The best exercise in the world is whichever one YOU will do!

Your body was meant to move. God did not intend for us to live a sedentary lifestyle. Our modern lifestyles have left us bereft of the daily movement that we need to maintain our health. We use the remote control rather than get up to change the TV channel. We drive our car from one store to another in the same shopping center. We take the elevator up one flight of stairs instead of walking. We sit in front of the computer at work for hours at a time only to come home and sit in front of the TV.

Two hundred years ago, humans did not need to exercise. The daily routine of farm life was rigorous enough that the body received a good workout for all of the muscle groups. With the start of the industrial revolution in the 1800s, machines began to replace the work that many humans used to do. As people began to migrate to the city in favor of factory work over farm work, natural exercise began to decline. With the invention of the automobile in the late 1800s, walking and cycling as the primary means of traveling short distances fell out of favor. The biggest hit to exercise came in the 1980s as TV viewing exploded with cable TV and video games. The availability of a wide array of viewing choices twenty-four hours a day replaced other, more active recreational pursuits. Video games replaced outdoor, interactive games for youths and adults alike.

Just about every adult knows that he or she needs to exercise. But according to Caroline Wilbert, a staff writer for WebMD, data from 2009 show that only about half of Americans exercise regularly, with regularly being defined as at least three sessions a week for thirty minutes at a time.

According to the A.C. Nielsen Co., the average American watches more than four hours of TV each day (or twenty-eight hours per week, or two months of nonstop TV-watching per year). In a sixty-five-year life, that person will have spent nine years glued to the tube. Professor Norman Herr, Ph.D., professor of science education at the California State University, Northridge, offers the following facts about TV viewing:

- Percentage of households that possess at least one television: 99
- Number of TV sets in the average U.S. household: 2.24
- Percentage of U.S. homes with three or more TV sets: 66
- Number of hours per day that TV is on in an average U.S. home: 6 hours, 47 minutes
- Percentage of Americans who regularly watch television while eating dinner: 66
- Number of hours of TV watched annually by Americans: 250 billion
- Value of that time assuming an average wage of $5/hour: $1.25 trillion
- Percentage of Americans who pay for cable TV: 56
- Number of videos rented daily in the U.S.: 6 million
- Number of public library items checked out daily: 3 million
- Percentage of Americans who say they watch too much TV: 49

The concept of creating a block of time in our daily schedules to exercise is really not a natural concept. Exercise should be a normal part of your daily routine. Never was this made clearer to me than when I was on a missions trip to Kenya in 1997. I was explaining to the daughter of one our hosts, a very gracious young lady who was about twenty-five, how I use a treadmill every day. She gave me a quizzical look and asked me to clarify what a treadmill was. As I did my best to explain a treadmill , she looked at me as if I were insane and said, "You mean you get on a machine and you pretend you are walking somewhere but you really are not going anywhere? Why not just get outside and walk?" I had no ready answer for her question.

Still, the reality of American life is that we *do* have to consciously work exercise into our daily routine.  As I stated above, the best exercise is the one you will do. So plan a fitness routine that fits with who you are and how you can best fit it in. Whatever routine you choose, strive to have a balance of weight bearing exercises, cardio exercises, resistance exercises, and flexibility exercises.

## WEIGHT-BEARING EXERCISES

Weight-bearing exercises are those exercises in which you have to use your legs to support the weight of your body. Weight-bearing exercises include walking, jumping rope, dancing, climbing stairs, kick boxing, hopping, and skipping. These exercises can also be good cardio exercises provided that they are done long enough and with enough intensity.

## CARDIO EXERCISES

Cardio exercises, also referred to as aerobic exercises, are those that elevate your heart rate for a certain period of time, at least twenty minutes. This provides benefits to your cardiovascular system and improves the overall condition of your body. In addition to the exercises listed under weight bearing, cycling and swimming are good cardio workouts.

## RESISTANCE EXERCISES

Resistance exercises are exercises in which your body is working against the force of another object. When this occurs, your body builds muscle mass and bone. Examples of resistance exercises are weights, resistance bands, and water.

Muscle mass on your body is highly desirable if you want to lose and maintain your weight. A pound of muscle and a pound of fat both weigh the same, but muscle is denser and it takes less space on your body. A good way to think of it is to compare a pound of steak to a pound of cheese puffs. The cheese puffs are lighter, so the container you will need for a pound of cheese puffs will be bigger than the one you will need to fit a pound of steak. If you compared two women of the same height, both weighing 150 pounds, the one who is lean and has good muscle mass will wear a dress size smaller than a woman who has a higher percentage of body fat.

Not only do toned muscles take up less space on your body, they burn more calories. Lean muscle mass is more biologically active than fat. Even at rest, your muscles will burn more calories than the fat tissue on your body. Lean muscle burns three times more calories than fat. This helps to boost your metabolism, which helps you to not only lose weight, but keep it off for good.

As you age, you lose lean muscle mass. The process of losing muscle mass is called sarcopenia. Research at Tufts has shown that from about the age of forty-five, the average person loses muscle mass at the rate of approximately 1 percent per year, rising to 1 percent to 2 percent from the age of fifty. By age seventy, a healthy person has 20 percent less muscle mass than he or she had at thirty-six, according to Science News (McMath). Everyone can benefit from adding resistance training to their fitness routine. However, if you are over age forty-five, it is imperative that you do so.

Many females are afraid to add strength training to their workout because they do not want to bulk up and look like Hulk Hogan. This is an unfounded fear. If you see a woman who is overly muscular, she is working very, very, very, hard so that her physique bulks up; her body did not get that way by lifting weights two to three times a week. Men easily bulk up because they have more testosterone than women, and testosterone is a key factor in muscle growth. But for a woman, lifting weights two to three times a week will yield a toned body that burns calories more efficiently.

## FLEXIBILITY EXERCISES

Flexibility exercises are those that help to keep the body flexible. These include yoga, Pilates and stretching routines. Yoga and Pilates can also help to tone your body and build lean muscle mass.

I vary my exercise routine based on the seasons, the weather, and my mood. Walking is my favorite weight-bearing activity. I walk at a rapid pace with the goal of doing four miles an hour. When it is too cold/snowy/rainy/windy to walk, I have a stationary bike that I ride for thirty minutes. Some days I put on my favorite musical DVD and dance for an hour, or access an exercise video from Exercise TV. I never stick to the same routine for longer than two weeks because I get bored quickly. However, I do know other people that do one activity, such as the treadmill, walking, stationary bike, or elliptical faithfully and they are able to stay toned and keep their weight in check.

I lift weights two to three times a week and vary the routine based on whether I am interspersing weight lifting with riding my bike, or following a routine from a DVD. Regardless of which exercise routine I choose, I end the routine with five minutes of stretching.

## BENEFITS OF EXERCISE

There are many benefits to exercise. First and foremost, exercise helps to control your weight. If you are sincere about being slim for life, you will need to make exercise a part of your lifestyle. The more active you are, the more calories your body will burn on a daily basis. Experts vary as to the amount of exercise that is optimal for good health. Some recommend thirty minutes a day and others recommend one hour. Gaining in popularity is the 10,000 steps advice, which computes to about five miles of walking a day.

Besides helping you to control your weight, there are other, lesser-known benefits of exercise. I once heard someone say that if all of the benefits of exercise could be marketed and put into a pill, it would be the number-one-selling pill on the market! Exercise can help manage and prevent many health conditions, such as high blood pressure, high cholesterol, depression, type 2 diabetes, arthritis, and even cancer.

Exercise can help you reduce stress and elevate your mood. When you exercise, your body releases chemicals called endorphins. Endorphins are your body's feel-good chemicals and are the same chemicals that are released in the body during orgasm. They will trigger a positive feeling in the body, not unlike that of morphine, and give you a sense of overall well-being. They can make you feel like you have arrived somewhere over the rainbow!

Exercise contributes to a positive self-esteem. Have you ever completed a task you had been putting off doing for while? Can you recall the sense of satisfaction and accomplishment that you felt from knowing you had finally gotten it done? When you exercise regularly you will get a sense of accomplishment and earn a great big pat on the back from yourself. It helps you to foster a "Yes I Can!" attitude.

Exercise helps you to sleep better, provided you do not do it right before bedtime. Exercising before bedtime will leave you feeling energized and awake, which is how you want to feel during your day, but not before bedtime. If you are exercising to promote better rest, it appears that the best time to do so is four to five hours before bedtime and to make the routine a cardio routine.

Exercise helps to build strong bones and ward off osteoporosis. Weight bearing, resistance, and flexibility exercises are good exercises to build strong bones.

## CREATIVE WAYS TO INCREASE YOUR ACTIVITY LEVEL

- Take the stairs whenever possible. I make it a rule to not take the elevator unless I am carrying something heavy or am ascending more than four floors.
- Take stair climbing breaks at work. When I worked in an office setting, I challenged myself to take stair breaks, where I would go up and down the stairs until I climbed 100 stairs at a time, and would do this three to five times a day. The staircase was outside my office door and one flight of stairs was twenty steps, so I would climb the staircase five times consecutively.
- Do push-ups using a counter/table/desk top or your car whenever you are waiting or transitioning. Doing just ten at a time will help to strengthen your arms.
- Park as far away from the entrance of the mall as you safely can. Refuse to drive around looking for the closest parking spot.
- If you ride the bus to work, purposely get off the bus a few blocks before your stop so you can walk the rest of the way.
- When in a shopping center and you have two stores to visit, park your car midway between the two stores and walk to both of them.
- Whenever you are standing in line for anything, exercise. Try contracting and releasing your stomach muscles or your gluteal muscle. If you do this enough times, you begin to feel the burn.
- Take as many phone calls as possible standing and marching in place, rather than sitting during the conversation.

# REFERENCES FOR CHAPTER FOUR

Mcmath, D. Livestrong. *How fast do you lose muscle mass?* Accessed January 20, 2012 at http://www.livestrong.com/article/289811-how-fast-do-you-lose-muscle-mass/#ixzz1fu49Cmid

Norman, H. *Television and Health. Source book for teaching science* Accessed November 18, 2011 at http://www.csun.edu/science/health/docs/tv&health.html

Oz. M. *What happens to my muscle mass at 40?* Accessed January 20, 2012 at http://www.sharecare.com/question/my-muscle-mass-at-40

# CHAPTER FIVE
# YOUR EXCITING NEW EATING PLAN

## THE HUNTER-GATHERER DIET

The basic principles of *How to Eat Yourself Slim and Never Diet Again* are based on what is known as the Hunter-Gatherer diet, which has also been referred to as the Paleolithic diet, the Stone Age diet, the Garden of Eden diet, and the Cave Man diet. Are you ready to run away now? Please don't go!

The Hunter-Gatherer diet is based on the diet of our ancestors over 10,000 years ago. Their basic diet consisted of what they hunted—animals and fowl—what they fished, and what they gathered—berries, nuts, seeds, vegetables, fruits, and roots.

Early humans did not eat a diet that consisted of grain products like we do today. Our modern diet contains lots of grains such as corn, wheat, and rice; many grain products that come from flour, such as bread and pasta; and other grain products such as cereals and oatmeal. Because grain products are so dense in carbohydrates, humans today consume many more calories than did our ancestors.

The Hunter-Gatherer diet is the basis for many popular diets today including the South Beach Diet, The Maker's Diet, The 17-Day Diet, the Zone Diet, and the Atkins Diet. All of these diets restrict the amount of carbohydrates you can consume while in the weight loss and maintenance phase. Some are more carbohydrate restrictive than others, but all of them are based on the same premise: the wrong type and the amount of carbohydrates in your diet is the cause of weight gain and are what prohibit you from losing weight.

## WHY CARBOHYDRATES MAKE YOU FAT

Excess Carbohydrates = Weight Gain. Whether the carbs are from bread, cereal, sugar, soda, beer, or fruit juice, eating too many carbs causes weight gain. All carbs, regardless of how they start out, get broken down in the body to the simple sugar called glucose. Some carbs are digested more rapidly than others, such as a sugary drink, a donut, or candy.

After you consume a high-carbohydrate meal, the glucose in your bloodstream rises rapidly. To deal with the excess glucose in your bloodstream, your pancreas must go to work to produce insulin in proportion to the amount of glucose in the blood stream so that it can be removed.

Insulin takes the glucose out of your bloodstream by first converting it into a starch called glycogen. Glycogen gets stored in the liver and in muscles. But just like the storeroom or the garage in your home that only can take so much stuff before you need to rent a storage space, the liver and muscles can only store so much glycogen and any excess glycogen is stored as body fat. This is how you gain weight.

Insulin is the hormone that is responsible for fat storage. Carbs produce an insulin response. Fats do not elicit an insulin response in your body and protein elicits a low insulin response in your body.

After a high-carbohydrate meal, your blood glucose level will return to normal in about ninety minutes. However, the insulin in your bloodstream is still very high. So although your blood glucose is normal, the insulin continues to store the glucose away in the form of fat. This causes your glucose level to fall below normal and guess what? You feel hungry all over again! And what do most people do when they are hungry? Eat! And if another high-carbohydrate meal is consumed, this vicious cycle continues. This is why excess carbs in your diet make you gain weight, and a weight-loss program that is high in carbs will result in slower weight loss.

## INSULIN RESISTANCE

Insulin resistance occurs when the cells in your body become resistant to the effects of insulin. This means that when your body produces insulin, the liver, muscle, and fat cells decrease their response to insulin, and glucose levels remain high in the blood. With glucose levels remaining high in the blood even more insulin is produced which means even more fat is stored. Insulin resistance is often a precursor to type II diabetes.

## LOSING WEIGHT VS. LOSING FAT

Have you ever seen the ads:

"Lose 10 pounds in 10 days!"

Can your body really lose weight that fast? Yes it can, but your body will not be losing fat. A football player on a hot day can lose ten pounds, and most of it will be just water. Crash diets will help you see a dip in the scale rapidly but this weight loss will not be permanent.

In order to lose weight permanently, you must start to burn the excess fat that is stored in your body. To help burn the excess fat, you must decrease your body's present supply of fuel from blood glucose. Translation: cut down on the carbs.

The editors at Diabetes Health explain it this way:

*When you eat carbs, your capacity to use fat is limited. Increasing blood glucose during dieting stimulates insulin release. Even at very low concentrations of insulin, fat synthesis is activated and break-up of fat is inhibited. This means that if you eat a carbohydrate-based low-fat diet, you force your body into a fat-making mode, not a fat-using mode.*

*Insulin inhibits the production of fat-burning enzymes, thereby preventing your body's fat cells from releasing their fat. This stops your body from burning your stored fat and makes it impossible for you to lose the weight you have put on.*

WebMd sheds some more light on why low-carbohydrate diets are effective:

*By restricting carbohydrates drastically to a mere fraction of that found in the typical American diet, the body goes into a different metabolic state called ketosis, whereby it burns its own fat for fuel. Normally the body burns carbohydrates for fuel -- this is the main source of fuel for your brain, heart, and many other organs. A person in ketosis is getting energy from ketones, little carbon fragments that are the fuel created by the breakdown of fat stores. When the body is in ketosis, you tend to feel less hungry, and thus you're likely to eat less than you might otherwise...*

*As a result, your body changes from a carbohydrate-burning engine into a fat-burning engine. So instead of relying on the carbohydrate-rich items you might typically consume for energy, and leaving your fat stores just where they were before (alas, the hips, belly, and thighs), your fat stores become a primary energy source.*

The Harvard School of Public Health reports that:

*Recent research provides reassurance that eating a lot of protein doesn't harm the heart. In fact, it is possible that eating more protein, especially vegetable protein, while cutting back on easily-digested carbohydrates may benefit the heart. A 20-year prospective study of 82,802 women found that those who ate low-carbohydrate diets that were high in vegetable sources of fat or protein had a 30 percent lower risk of heart disease, compared with women who ate high-carbohydrate, low-fat diets. But women who ate low-carbohydrate diets that were high in animal fats or proteins did not have a reduced risk of heart disease.*

There are concerns about high-protein diets putting stress on the kidneys and liver. Lisa Zerasky, registered dietician at the Mayo Clinic, explains that a high-protein diet may cause or worsen liver or kidney problems because your body may already have trouble eliminating all the waste products of protein metabolism. She is quick to add, however, that for most healthy people, a high-protein diet generally isn't harmful if followed for a short time, such as three to four months, and may help with weight loss.

## THE DOWNSIDE OF SEVERELY RESTRICTING CARBS

Many weight loss programs severely restrict carbs in the initial phase. While this will help the number on the scale to decrease faster, there is a downside to having a very low level of carbs in your diet.

Your brain loves glucose and is constantly searching for glucose as fuel. Glucose is your brain's preferred source of energy. With a very low level of carbs in your diet, you may find it hard to concentrate and you may even get a headache.

Eating carbs raises serotonin levels in your brain. Serotonin is a neurotransmitter that is involved in the transmission of nerve impulses and is known as the "feel good" chemical. It helps us to relax and have a general feeling of well-being. This is why so many high carbohydrate foods are called "comfort foods." Severely restricting carbs may make you feel irritable and jittery. Trying to keep a positive attitude about weight loss while you are physically feeling irritable is hard to do.

Severely restricting carbs means that most of your diet will be protein and fat. Without added fiber in the diet, constipation may result and you may feel bloated and uncomfortable.

## MY EXPERIENCE WITH REDUCING CARBS

For years my family knew that I had FMS Syndrome—Feed Me Soon! Whenever I was hungry it was a chronic condition and one that had to be dealt with quickly. If I didn't eat right away, irritability would set in, I could not focus, I felt faint, and I would even get slight tremors in my hands.

In 2004, I was about ten pounds heavier than I wanted to be. I am 5'8" and have a medium frame. According to the height and weight chart included in this book, my healthy weight is between 136 – 150 pounds. The weight that I feel best at is 146 pounds. I heard about the South Beach Diet and was interested in it because it promised to take off six to nine pounds in just two weeks and that I would lose belly fat first.

The South Beach Diet is a low-carbohydrate diet and during the first two weeks, no fruit or grain products were allowed. I was a little alarmed by the lack of fiber from the no grains and the no fruit requirement for the first two weeks, but I decided to give a try. To deal with the lack of fiber I took a mild laxative.

My results were life changing but not because I lost six to nine pounds. I only lost five. But what I did lose was the FMS Syndrome. The diet apparently stabilized my insulin levels and I no longer felt like I was in dire straits whenever I was hungry. I also began to notice how much clearer my mind felt without all the sugar coursing through my bloodstream. These were unexpected results but ones for which I was grateful.

Since my experience with the South Beach Diet, I monitor the amount of starchy carbs from grains that I consume throughout the day and in any one meal. Most of my carbs come from fruit, vegetables, beans and legumes. Grains based carbs such as bread, pasta, and rice I eat in small portions and no longer consume them everyday.   This keeps me closest to my ideal weight.

## EAT YOURSELF SLIM EATING PLAN

From my own personal experience and the experience of others, I am convinced that the fastest and most pleasant way to weight loss is to restrict, *but not eliminate*, carbohydrates in the diet. I prefer this way because I am not consumed with cutting calories, portion control, or writing what I eat in a journal. I can eat until I feel satisfied, and have a snack if I feel hungry. I have fewer periods in the day when I experience an energy dip due to the swings in my insulin levels.

Since we all know that one of the biggest lies ever told was "one size fits all," *The Eat Yourself Slim Plan*  is not a one-size-fits-all eating plan. The level of carbohydrate restriction as you are in the weight loss phase is an individual choice. You may find that you can handle no grain and no fruit without feeling irritable. Or you may be able to adjust to a having a few servings of low-sugar fruits like berries and apples per day. Or you may need to add a carbohydrate like beans, which will give you a carb boost and added fiber.

While the eating plan is not one size fits all, there are certain principles that you will follow that hopefully will become lifestyle principles. The knowledge that you gained in this book regarding how certain foods damage your health should be incorporated into how you eat daily, regardless of whether or not you are trying to lose weight. This is the secret to eating yourself slim and never dieting again: you permanently change your eating habits so that your body will remain slim. Even though I can experience a few pounds of weight gain as a result of a vacation, eating took many traditional holiday dishes around Christmas, an injury where I cannot exercise, or not being careful about the number of carbs I am consuming, the few pounds are still within my average weight range and my waist circumference remains below 35". I purposely strive to keep my weight just a few pounds below the upper end for my height so I have a few pounds to play with.

Here are the ten principles that you will follow on the Eat Yourself Slim plan:

1. Eliminate white foods from your diet: white flour, white bread, white rice, white sugar (brown sugar is white sugar with molasses, so it is still white sugar and needs to be eliminated). White potatoes, because they are so high on the glycemic index which causes an insulin surge in your body, should be eaten sparingly. Any fruit or vegetable that is white, like cauliflower, is still a healthy choice for you.

2. Eliminate trans fat in the form of partially hydrogenated and hydrogenated oils from your diet. This should be eliminated 100 percent. Once a food is fried in oil, it becomes a trans fat. Fried foods must be a rarity, consumed no more than once a month in a very small quantity. Fried foods include foods like potato chips, donuts, and corn chips (yes, corn chips are fried; look for the baked ones in the supermarket).

3. Eliminate/severely curtail processed foods from your diet. Eat everything as close to how it occurs naturally as possible. If you do not know what an ingredient is in a food, do not eat it. Processed foods include lunchmeat, bacon, frozen food entrees, snack foods, etc.

4. Eliminate high fructose corn syrup and artificial sweeteners from your diet.

5. Beverages: Drink a minimum of 64 ounces of water every day. Go for antioxidant-rich green tea in your diet daily.

6. Fiber: Consume 25 grams or more of fiber every day from natural grains, fruits, and vegetables.

7. Protein: Aim for 75 to 100 grams of protein daily from lean cuts of meat, lean white-meat poultry without the skin, and fish; substitute legumes and beans for protein instead of animal foods. Eat oily fish like salmon and tuna a minimum of twice a week.

8. Fruits and vegetables: Eat a minimum of four servings of fruit and five servings of vegetables every day. Remember that a serving is one-half of a cup of fruit or cooked vegetables, and two cups of leafy raw vegetables. One medium-sized pear is two servings of fruit. Doing this may appear to be difficult at first glance, but it is easier than you think once you begin to eliminate the unhealthy foods from your diet.

9. Carbohydrates: Limit grain servings from breads, oats, etc. to four servings per day.
10. Fat: Include 2–3 servings daily of omega 3 fats in your diet from olive oil, flax seeds, and chia seeds. Limit saturated fat found in dairy and other animal products to 20 grams per day.

Now that I have told you what to eliminate, I am going to free you from any guilt when you do eat foods that are on the elimination list. I acknowledge that you are on a dual journey. You purchased this book because you want to be slim for life; your intent may not have been to eat healthy. For many of you, doing both simultaneously will be a challenge. If you find that the adjustment to healthy eating during the weight loss phase makes you feel deprived and you would rather substitute something that I recommend you eliminate, then allow yourself to eat it. If you find yourself resisting food, this may result in your feeling deprived which is not a positive state to be in. The goal is for you to learn enough about good food that you will crave to eat healthy food rather than unhealthy food. The goal is for you to start humming to yourself a song about positive eating or saying an affirmation that makes healthy food appealing.

While I am acknowledging that there will be times when less-than-optimum nutrition will enter your body, I am not advocating that you eat whatever you want in moderation. This concept is a scary one because there is no true definition of what eating unhealthy foods in moderation is. Everyone brings his or her own definition. I have watched people eat unhealthy food day in and day out and believe that they only eat unhealthy foods in moderation. They believe this because they are not eating the same food every day. So one day they eat fried chicken wings, the next a ham and cheese biscuit sandwich for breakfast, and the next day pizza for dinner. They may not be eating the same food every day, but they are eating lots of unhealthy food.

For the benefit of your health and so you will not slip back into unhealthy eating patterns, once you have reached your target weight, learn to limit the amounts and frequency of the foods that are on the elimination list. My strategy is to limit it to no more than once per week and most weeks I eat nothing on the elimination list. Two items I never knowingly consume are partially hydrogenated oil and high fructose corn syrup. If I am a guest at someone's home I do not query them about what is in the food. I know where these ingredients might be and just choose other foods. I eat what is set before me with thanksgiving and do not get weird about it. I already know that most catered meals are adulterated so I no longer eat much at social functions. I choose as wisely as I can when at a restaurant or on vacation. Fried foods I limit to rare occasions, and I probably eat them no more than nine times per year.

## PHASE ONE OF EAT YOURSELF SLIM: DAY 1–15

There are three levels to follow in phase one and they correspond to the number of carbohydrates that you will choose to eat on a daily basis. Phase one is designed to accelerate your weight loss. With the recommended level of restricted carbs, you should lose 3 to 4 pounds per week. The more you restrict carbohydrates, the faster you will lose weight and the faster your sugar cravings will go away. You may choose to begin your first week with level one, and then switch to level two or level three for your second week. You can also choose to switch the levels from one day to the next.

*Level One*

Protein: Unlimited amounts of the following protein. Remember that animal sources of protein contain saturated fat, so stick with the leanest cuts of meat possible. During this phase you will probably exceed the daily recommended amount of saturated fat. This will just be temporary and not a style of eating that you will want to continue once you approach your ideal weight.

- Beef: Lean cuts of beef such as flank steak, top sirloin steak, or lean ground beef with fat drained.
- Poultry: Baked or broiled chicken and turkey breast with the skin removed, no-salt turkey lunchmeat (this is minimally processed lunchmeat and the only one that I recommend), low-fat turkey and chicken sausages, lean ground turkey or chicken.
- Fish: All types. Keep in mind that shellfish are high in cholesterol.
- Dairy: Cheese, eggs.

Non-starchy vegetables: Unlimited amounts of artichoke, asparagus, bamboo shoots, bean sprouts, broccoli, Brussels sprouts, cabbage (green, bok choy, Chinese), cauliflower, celery, cucumber, daikon, eggplant, green beans, greens (collard, kale, mustard, turnip), hearts of palm, Italian beans, jicama, kohlrabi, leeks, mushrooms, okra, onions, pea pods, peppers, radishes, rutabaga, salad greens, sprouts, snap peas, Swiss chard, tomato, turnips, water chestnuts, wax beans, and zucchini.

Added Fats: Two tablespoons of oil/salad dressing.

Nuts: Limit to one serving per day in exchange for a tablespoon of fat.

*Level Two*

Eat all the foods in level one, adding the following for a few more carbs in your diet:

- One or two ½-cup servings of plain cottage cheese or plain yogurt daily. To make the cottage cheese or plain yogurt enjoyable, mix with a low-sugar fruit. This is an excellent snack to eat between meals.
- Fruit: one to two ½-cup servings of low-sugar fruit. Low-sugar fruits include all berries, apples, oranges, peaches, grapes, pears, and grapefruit.

*Level Three*

Eat all the foods in level one and level two, choosing only one ½-cup serving of fruit per day, and one ½-cup serving of cottage cheese or yogurt per day, and choosing <u>one</u> of the following starches per day.

- Legumes: ½ cup daily of legumes: black beans, kidney beans, split peas, lentils, garbanzo beans, navy beans, and lima beans.
- ½ cup of starchy vegetables: sweet potatoes, corn, yams, lima beans, squash, carrots, turnips, peas, and beets.

*Snacks for Phase One*

- Low-fat mozzarella cheese sticks.
- ½ cup yogurt with mixed fruit.
- Turkey breast roll-ups with Swiss cheese.

*Condiments*

Tomato-based salsa, hot sauce, mustard, small amounts of fat-free dressings, small amounts of fat-free sour cream, and lite soy sauce. Low-sugar ketchup is available, but it is sweetened with artificial sweeteners. Use sparingly, if at all.

*Beverages*

Enjoy green tea or herbal tea sweetened with stevia. The more water you drink, the better. Water helps to flush the fat out of your system and helps you not retain water weight. Coffee contains caffeine, unless you are drinking decaf, and the caffeine can act as an appetite suppressant and a diuretic, and can even boost your metabolism a little. If you are used to drinking coffee, continue using a small amount of cream or milk if you do not drink it black (coffee creamers contain a host of chemicals and some contain trans fat).

To help boost your metabolism, you will want to add a broth from kombu seaweed to your diet daily. According to Dr. Oz and other health practitioners, kombu is important in the diet because of its high content of iodine, a trace mineral that is essential to regulating our thyroid gland. Our thyroid gland produces two hormones that control metabolism. Our bodies do not make iodine so we must get it from food. Also, there is a pigment in kombu called fucoxanthin, which may boost production of a protein involved in fat metabolism.

Kombu comes in long, thick, brown strips and you can purchase it from health food stores. To make a broth, use one strip of kombu. Rinse it first then cut it up and put it in four cups of water. Cook it over low heat for about thirty minutes. Drink one cup per day. If the broth is not to your liking, you may use it as a stock for soup.

*Fiber Supplements*

Depending on the type of vegetables you eat, you may find that your diet is lacking in fiber without any fiber from whole grains during phase one. Hence, you may want to consider a fiber supplement. I recommend that you use Metamucil Clear and Natural or Nature's Sunshine Psyllium Hulls. Use these products according to package instructions and make sure you are drinking the recommended amount of water. Unlike a laxative, fiber supplements do not artificially stimulate your system for a bowel movement to occur and are not habit forming.

*Breakfast During Phase One*

For many people, managing their lunch and dinner during phase one is relatively easy. Breakfast seems to be the biggest challenge, where eggs seem to be the only option. Below is a week of suggestions to keep your breakfasts interesting and tasty.

Day One: Scrambled eggs and natural chicken sausage.

Day Two: Veggie and cheese omelet.

Day Three and Four: Spinach and mushroom quiche without crust. This is a two-day breakfast because the quiche usually lasts for two days.

Day Five: Two boiled eggs and natural turkey sausage.

Day Six: Salmon cakes.

Day Seven: Southwestern omelet with ground turkey seasoned with taco seasoning.

## PHASE TWO OF EAT YOURSELF SLIM: DAY 16–30

During this phase as you are increasing the carbohydrates in your diet, your weight loss will slow down. Weight loss of 2 to 3 pounds per week should be expected in this phase.

*Level One*

Eat all of the foods from phase one level one adding the following:

- One to two ½-cup servings of cottage cheese or plain yogurt per day.
- One to two ½-cup servings of low-sugar fruit.
- ½ cup of legumes OR ½ cup of starchy vegetables: sweet potatoes, corn, yams, lima beans, squash, carrots, turnips, peas, and beets.

*Level Two*

Eat all the foods from phase one level two adding the following:
- ½ cup of legumes per day OR ½ cup of starchy vegetables.

*Level Three*

Eat all the foods from phase one level three, with the following modifications:

- One to two ½-cup servings of cottage cheese or plain yogurt per day.
- One to two ½-cup servings of low-sugar fruit per day.
- ½-cup serving of starchy vegetables.

- ½-cup of legumes OR ½-cup serving of grains: brown rice, quinoa, amaranth, barley, bulgur, bran, old-fashioned oats (not the instant kind in a package).

## PHASE THREE OF EAT YOURSELF SLIM: DAY 31 AND BEYOND

If continued accelerated weight loss is your goal, you should continue on phase two, level three until you reach your ideal weight.

If continued weight loss at a slower pace is your goal, you can begin on day 31 to ease whole grains back into your diet and eat a wider variety of fruits. Now that increased carbohydrates are in your diet, you must begin to pay attention to portion sizes and overall calorie consumption. Your weight loss will be accelerated or decelerated based on many how calories you consume, how many carbs you eat, how much you exercise, and how much muscle you build (remember muscle burns more calories than fat).

Your daily eating plan should be one that keeps you satisfied without you constantly thinking about food or your next meal. It is recommended that you focus on eating five times a day—three meals and two snacks. The number of calories that should be consumed is different for each person, based on the person's ideal weight. You must determine how many calories you need in your daily diet to maintain your ideal weight. You can calculate your caloric needs at my website www.eatyourslimandneverdietagain.com

For many, many, many (did I say many?) people, just focusing on eating good, healthy food is enough to shed unwanted pounds. Without all of the unhealthy food in the diet, maintaining an ideal weight comes naturally. However, even healthy food can make you gain weight if you eat in excess. This is especially true when it comes to consuming too many whole-grain products.

For most people 1,400 calories a day with exercise will result in losing 1–2 pounds per week. On the next page is an example of 1,400 calories a day while meeting all of the requirements on the *Eat Yourself Slim* plan.

## 1,400 Calories a Day Plan

| | Cal | Protein | Fib | Fat | Whole Grain | Fruit | Vegetable | Dairy |
|---|---|---|---|---|---|---|---|---|
| **Snack for workout** | | | | | | | | |
| 3 ounces yogurt, ½ banana | 50 / 55 | 9 | 1.5 | | | 1 | | .5 |
| **Breakfast** | | | | | | | | |
| 6 ounces plain Greek yogurt, 1 cup strawberries, | 100 / 77 | 18 | 5 | | | 2 | | 1.5 |
| 1 slice whole wheat toast, 1 tablespoon cream cheese | 80 / 50 | 4 | 3 | .5 | 1 | | | |
| **Lunch** | | | | | | | | |
| Soup containing beans and vegetables, one ounce of almonds | 200 / 162 | 9 / 6 | 9 / 3 | 1 | | | 3 | |
| **Snack** | | | | | | | | |
| Peanut butter and jelly, bread | 100 / 20 / 80 | 4 / 4 | 2 / 3 | .5 | 1 | | | |

| Dinner | | | | | | | | |
|---|---|---|---|---|---|---|---|---|
| 6 ounces baked tilapia, | 216 | 42 | | | | | | |
| 1½ cups cleansing vegetables, | 68 | 3 | 3 | | | | 3 | |
| ½ cup brown rice | 124 | 2 | 2 | | 1 | | | |
| TOTALS | 1382 | 100 | 32.5 | 2 | 3 | 3 | 6 | 2 |

## MY PERSONAL EATING PLAN

I have crafted an anti-inflammatory, low-cholesterol, high-fiber, low-sodium diet for my own nutritional needs that comes to about 2,200 calories per day. Overall, this is what I do:

1. Eat fish at least three times a week. Fish choices are wild caught salmon, light tuna, tilapia, and river trout. I do not eat shellfish. I steer clear of farm-raised fish with the exception of tilapia.
2. Poultry no more than twice a week, beef maybe once a month. I do not eat pork. Between the poultry and fish, I eat flesh foods no more than seven times a week. This is different from many people who eat them at every meal. I limit my consumption of animal flesh because of my genetic propensity towards high cholesterol.
3. Two to three servings of dairy daily. I use plain Greek yogurt and sweeten it with berries or a banana. I eat low-fat cheese for snacks, and use whole-milk cheese in dishes that I prepare.
4. Three to four servings of fruits daily.
5. Minimum of five servings of vegetables daily. These servings come easily with a large salad in the summer, or vegetable soups in the winter. I make sure I have at least two servings of a power vegetable daily. Power vegetables are the ones highest on the anti-inflammatory rating scale, such as kale, collards, and sweet potatoes.
6. Four servings of whole grains.
7. Beans/legumes five to seven times a week.

8. Three servings of good fats per day. This can be in the form of a serving of nuts (raw almonds and walnuts are my two favorites), peanut butter, tahini, olive oil, flax oil, chia seeds, flax seeds, or avocado.
9. Dessert once a week, no more than 300 calories.
10. Lots of water.

Eating healthy is a lifestyle. The benefits to your health are tremendous, not to mention how much better you will feel physically and mentally. Like any new habit or skill, it will feel strange at first. However, the more you practice it, the easier it becomes.

You now have the knowledge to begin your forty day journey to eating yourself slim and never dieting again. Your "bags" are packed with good groceries and your "passport" (which is this book) is in your hand. Your mind is made up, so get ready to set sail!

## REFERENCES FOR CHAPTER FIVE

Harvard School of Public Health. *The Nutrition Source.* Accessed January 31, 2012 at http://www.hsph.harvard.edu/nutritionsource/questions/protein-questions/

WebMd. *High protein, low carb diets.* Accessed February 24, 2012 at http://women.webmd.com/guide/high-protein-low-carbohydrate-diets

Zeratsky, K. *Are high-protein diets safe for weight loss?* Accessed February 24, 2012 at http://www.mayoclinic.com/health/high-protein-diets/AN00847

# CHAPTER SIX
# YOUR 40-DAY JOURNEY BEGINS

It is now time to begin your journey to a slimmer you. Imagine that in just forty days, you will have a new mindset toward eating and have the power and the tools to be as slim as you like forever!

During your forty-day journey, you will have a daily scripture reading and say aloud a new prayer every day for five days. On days six and seven, you will review the scriptures and prayers of the previous week. The rationale for this is that for some reason, people start diets on Monday, so the five prayers are designed to read Monday through Friday. On the weekends, when people tend to have a little more time, that is when all five prayers are to be read. Read your prayers aloud with emotion, sincerity, and passion. It is well known that whatever we say with emotion will be more readily picked up by our subconscious and transferred into a belief, as opposed to just reading the words in a flat monotone.

It is a good idea to say the prayer upon arising in the morning, in the evening before bedtime, and several times throughout the day. The more frequently you repeat these prayers, the faster you will develop the belief.

There is also space included for you to write your thoughts, prayers, emotions, challenges, etc. each day. There is something very powerful and effective about writing what you are feeling, so please allow yourself to participate in this process.

You will also have a weekly assignment. Just like the assignments you were given in chapter two, these assignments are an integral part of your success. Do not skip them! Make the time to complete them sometime during the week. The assignments do not have to be done at the beginning of the week, just as long as they are completed within the seven-day period.

It is assumed that you have already settled on which low-carbohydrate eating plan you will follow for the next forty days. The first day of your new eating plan should correspond with the prayer identified for day one.

## WEEK ONE ASSIGNMENT

Create a dream board filled with pictures of a slimmer you. A dream board will help you to visualize yourself slimmer and is just one more tool that will help you develop the mindset that it takes to be slim forever. A dream board can be any size or shape. I personally like using the tri-fold board that students use for science fair projects. This type of board can stand on its own anywhere and it gives lots of space to place blow up pictures and write big letters on it.

Put your name at the top of board with big, bold colorful letters. Under your name write something great about yourself like "I am beautiful, I am amazing, I am powerful," etc. Also write on the board at the top your ideal dress/jacket/pants size. At the bottom of the board, write the date by which you have decided you will achieve this goal.

Fill the board with pictures of you when you were slimmer. Add some of the nice outfits that you see online or in magazines that you would like to wear when you are slimmer. If you have an outfit (or two or three) that you just cannot give away because you have always believed that you would fit back into it, take a picture of the outfit(s) and put it on the board. Put this board in a place where you can see it every day. The more you see it, the better.

In addition to completing your dream board, reading your scripture, and saying the prayer aloud every day, practice your affirmations (created in chapter two) a minimum of twice a day. Add new ones if you can.

And keep on singing!

**DAY ONE**

*I can do all things through Christ who strengthens me.*
Philippians 4:13 (NKJV)

Dear God:

I thank you for new beginnings! Through the power of the Holy Spirit, I celebrate that I can do all things through Christ who strengthens me. I praise You that you have given me power over my thoughts. Today I choose to think joyous thoughts of how much You love me, how much You care for me, and how much You desire that I live an abundant life. I am excited that part of that abundant life is honoring my temple through wise choices in food and drink. I am so grateful that You are with me every step of the way as I embrace healthier eating habits that will result in me being slim for life. I am changing to Your glory!

_____
_____
_____
_____
_____
_____
_____
_____
_____
_____
_____
_____
_____
_____
_____
_____
_____
_____

## DAY TWO

*⁶Do not be anxious about anything, but in every situation, by prayer
and petition, with thanksgiving, present your requests to God.
⁷ And the peace of God, which transcends all understanding,
will guard your hearts and your minds in Christ Jesus.*
Philippians 4:6–7 (NIV)

Dear God:

As I begin my journey to eating myself slim, I embrace Your word, which tells me to not be anxious. I pray today with thanksgiving that you will empower me with everything I need to be successful in eating to be slim. I present my request today knowing that You will give me the courage and the mindset to move forward with conviction and ease. I reaffirm today that I can do all things through Christ who strengthens me. I pray for your peace as I change my mindset and eating habits. I know You will guard my heart and mind from thinking of unhealthy food and will help me to focus on eating well.

_____

_____

_____

_____

_____

_____

_____

_____

_____

_____

_____

_____

_____

_____

## DAY THREE

*But Daniel purposed in his heart that he would not defile himself with the portion of the king's delicacies, nor with the wine which he drank; therefore he requested of the chief of the eunuchs that he might not defile himself.[11] So Daniel said to the steward…,*
*[12] "Please test your servants for ten days, and let them give us vegetables to eat and water to drink.[13] Then let our appearance be examined before you, and the appearance of the young men who eat the portion of the king's delicacies; and as you see fit, so deal with your servants." [14] So he consented with them in this matter, and tested them ten days.[15] And at the end of ten days their features appeared better and fatter in flesh than all the young men who ate the portion of the king's delicacies.[16] Thus the steward took away their portion of delicacies and the wine that they were to drink, and gave them vegetables.*
Daniel 1:8, 11–16 (NKJV)

Dear God:

How great and excellent are you Lord in all the earth! The earth is filled with Your goodness and love. I am amazed by how every little detail of my life You have provided for. You gave me an abundance of fruits and vegetables to eat so that I could keep my body healthy. The natural anti-oxidants found in fruits and vegetables help protect my body from a host of diseases. The natural fiber in whole foods helps to eliminate toxins from my body. Now that I know this, the thought of eating sugary snacks, fried snacks, white flour snacks, and salty snacks have lost their appeal. Now when I want a snack, I reach into Your pantry—nature's pantry—and enjoy nourishing my body and brain. You have truly given me everything I need for life and godliness, and I thank you!

## DAY FOUR

> <sup>6</sup> *Do not eat the bread of a miser,*
> *Nor desire his delicacies;*
> <sup>7</sup> *For as he thinks in his heart, so is he.*
> *"Eat and drink!" he says to you,*
> *But his heart is not with you.*
> <sup>8</sup> *The morsel you have eaten, you will vomit up,*
> *And waste your pleasant words.*
> Proverbs 23:6–7 (NKJV)

Dear God:

I praise you for this new day! Each day is an opportunity to grow more into the image of Christ. As I choose to focus my thoughts today, I am reminded that Your word says that as a man thinks in his heart so is he. Today I think of myself as a person who is in total control of my eating habits. I am enjoying smaller portions and am learning to eat to live rather than live to eat. The promise of living a healthy, abundant life is very exciting and I am moving forward with joy and anticipation!

_____

_____

_____

_____

_____

_____

_____

_____

_____

_____

_____

_____

_____

_____

## DAY FIVE

> [23] *This is the LORD's doing; it is marvelous in our eyes.*
> [24] *This is the day which the LORD hath made;*
> *we will rejoice and be glad in it.*
> [25] *Save now, I beseech thee, O LORD: O LORD,*
> *I beseech thee, send now prosperity.*
> Psalms 118:23–25 (NKJV)

Dear God:

This is the day that You have made and I will rejoice and be glad in it! This is an exciting day for continued change for me. I am dissolving stale, archaic, outdated, unproductive, and unhealthy thoughts about how I feed my body, and replacing them with new, fresh, exhilarating, empowering, and healthy thoughts that are leading to my goal of a healthy weight and a healthy body. This process is so exciting that I greet each day with anticipation and joy. I know that the more I affirm my new thoughts and habits, the more they become a part of who I am. Thank you, Lord, for the power to change!

_____

_____

_____

_____

_____

_____

_____

_____

_____

_____

_____

_____

_____

_____

_____

_____

_____

## DAY SIX AND SEVEN

Read over the five passages from the previous week. Record your thoughts and insights here.

_____

_____

_____

_____

_____

_____

_____

_____

_____

_____

_____

_____

_____

_____

_____

_____

_____

_____

_____

_____

_____

_____

_____

_____

_____

_____

_____

_____

_____

_____

_____

_____

_____

_____

## WEEK TWO ASSIGNMENT

You have already begun to tap into the power of your subconscious as you take this joyful journey to a slender body. The daily affirmations, the songs, and remembering the details of your past successes are helping you to make the change to healthy eating habits. You will now elicit support from your subconscious mind even more by tapping into the amazing power of visualization.

Visualization is simply the practice of using your imagination to see something that you want in the future. We use the process of visualization often without really knowing it. Have you ever found yourself planning a vacation and imagined yourself lying on the beach soaking up the sun? Or what about looking forward to a long, hot bath after an exhausting day and you could feel yourself relax just thinking about how good the hot water would feel on your aching muscles?

When we focus our creative energies to see something that we want in the future, this communicates a strong message to the subconscious mind that causes a person to take action to make sure the object of her desire comes true. Some believers like to think of visualization as the personification of Hebrews 11:1: *"Faith is the confidence that what we hope for will actually happen; it gives us assurance about things we cannot see."* (NLT). By faith, you will begin to see yourself in a slim body.

For the next thirty-three days, or until you reach your ideal weight, take five minutes to focus your attention on what you look like slim. Sit in a quiet place where you will not be interrupted. It is beneficial to have as many associations with this situation as possible. Burn the same fragrant candle or incense, have the same soft music playing in the background, cover yourself with the same blanket, etc. Clear your mind and see yourself slender. Once you have an image of yourself slender, see you in your slender body interacting with people that you know. Create different scenes where you are interacting with a variety of people: on the beach, dancing, giving a talk, shopping for clothes, family gatherings, church, etc. Allow yourself to feel the joy and the excitement of interacting with others in your new, slim body.

Practice your affirmations every day. Add new ones if you can.

And keep on singing!

## DAY EIGHT

*⁵ Get wisdom! Get understanding!*
*Do not forget, nor turn away from the words of my mouth.*
*⁶ Do not forsake her, and she will preserve you;*
*Love her, and she will keep you.*
*⁷ Wisdom is the principal thing;*
*Therefore get wisdom.*
*And in all your getting, get understanding.*
Proverbs 4:5–7 (NKJV)

Dear God:

Thank you today for the knowledge You have placed in my path. As I am growing in my knowledge of how to feed my body so that I will be slim for life, I thank You that my understanding is increasing as well. It has been said that wisdom is knowledge applied. I am fully committed to applying the knowledge that I have learned, to strive to understand it better each day, and to walk in wisdom. My new eating habits are not only delightful; they will preserve my health and keep my body in great shape. Yes, it was wise of me to start this journey, and I will be even wiser at the end of it. Thank you, God, for wisdom!

---
---
---
---
---
---
---
---
---
---
---

## DAY NINE

*<sup>13</sup> For You formed my inward parts;*
*You covered me in my mother's womb.*
*<sup>14</sup>I will praise You, for I am fearfully and wonderfully made,*
*Marvelous are Your works,*
*And that my soul knows very well.*
*<sup>15</sup> My frame was not hidden from You,*
*When I was made in secret,*
*And skillfully wrought in the lowest parts of the earth.*
*Psalm 119:13–15 (NKJV)*

Dear God:

I praise You today, for I am fearfully and wonderfully made! You have made me a unique creation and there is no one else in the world that is a copy of me. I am an original! And since I am an original, today I choose original thoughts of the healthy and slim me that I am growing towards. The thoughts and ideas of advertisers who promote that eating unhealthy food in copious amounts is fun are mere rubbish to me, and those messages I ignore. My thoughts are focused on the original, beautiful, healthy me that You created. You made me an original; living my life as a carbon copy is unthinkable!

_____

_____

_____

_____

_____

_____

_____

_____

_____

_____

_____

_____

## DAY TEN

*⁶ Therefore I remind you to stir up the gift of God which
is in you through the laying on of my hands.
⁷ For God has not given us a spirit of fear, but
of power and of love and of a sound mind.*

*I Timothy 1:6–7 (NKJV)*

Dear God:

I greet this day with a song of praise! As I experience fresh breath in my nostrils that fills my lungs with air, I am grateful for the amazing body that You have created. I thank You for all of the things that work well in my body. I know my body will function optimally as I continue to consume good food that nourishes all of my organs and cells. It is so exciting to eat in a way that honors and protects my health. I thank you for a sound mind that has allowed me to make wise choices. I can feel Your spirit encouraging me and leading me every step of the way! I know today will be another successful day of eating to be slim for life!

_____

_____

_____

_____

_____

_____

_____

_____

_____

_____

_____

_____

_____

_____

## DAY ELEVEN

*Stand fast therefore in the liberty by which Christ has made us free,*
*and do not be entangled again with a yoke of bondage.*
Galatians 5:1 (NKJV)

Dear God:

Your word tells me to stand fast in the liberty by which Christ has made me free and not be entangled again with a yoke of bondage. I am grateful that I have freedom in all areas of my life to make wise choices. I am exhilarated that I have made wise choices regarding my eating habits for the past ten days. I know this is just the beginning, but the past ten days give me proof that I can control what I choose to eat. I declare and confirm that I have broken the yoke of bondage of being a constant slave to food. I celebrate my freedom from old, useless eating habits. I am eating a new way now. It feels so good to be free and in control!

_____
_____
_____
_____
_____
_____
_____
_____
_____
_____
_____
_____
_____
_____
_____
_____
_____
_____

## DAY TWELVE

*Now the Lord is the Spirit; and where the Spirit of
the Lord is, there is freedom.*
2 Corinthians 3:17 (NIV)

Dear God:

Your word tells me that *"The Lord is the Spirit, and where the Spirit of the Lord is, there is freedom."* I thank you, Lord, for Your spirit that dwells in me and the freedom of choice You have given me. Today I marvel in the wonderful freedom I have in choosing my thoughts and actions. The more I affirm my desire to have better health, healthy eating habits, and a slim body, the freer I am to make food choices consistent with my desires. I am thankful that I have the discretion to eat when and what I determine I want to eat, rather than responding to food that is in a room. I am confident in turning down offers of food. I am secure in ignoring any disparaging comments regarding why I am choosing to eat differently. I am walking in food freedom!

_____

_____

_____

_____

_____

_____

_____

_____

_____

_____

_____

_____

_____

_____

_____

_____

_____

_____

## DAY THIRTEEN AND FOURTEEN

Read over the five prayers of this week. Go back and re-read some of your favorites from week one. Record your thoughts and insights here.

_____
_____
_____
_____
_____
_____
_____
_____
_____
_____
_____
_____
_____
_____
_____
_____
_____
_____
_____
_____
_____
_____
_____
_____
_____
_____
_____

## WEEK THREE ASSIGNMENT

Write a narrative of what happens when you slide into a great outfit that is your ideal dress/jacket/pants size. Describe the outfit (this may be an outfit you already have, one you invent in your mind, or one you have seen while shopping). Describe every detail of the outfit. Tell to which event you are wearing the outfit. Give as many details of the event as possible.

- What is the date of the event?
- What type of event is it?
- Is a choir singing?
- Is a band playing?
- Is it a red carpet event?
- How will you arrive?
- Are you arriving solo, with a date, or with a group of friends?
- Is it an outdoor affair?
- Is the room illuminated with bright or dim lights?
- Is it lit with candles?
- Who will you see at this event?
- Whose eyes will pop when they see your slim figure?
- What are some of the comments you can hear them saying?
- How does it make you feel? Describe your feelings in detail.

You can take this a little further (and maybe even save some time) by recording it. Using your webcam or camera on your mobile device, record yourself telling the story. Delight in your feelings and allow your excitement to show. Hearing yourself say this aloud helps to cement the image of the new you deep in your subconscious and your mind will go to work to make sure that it will come to pass.

Review your story every day this week. Enjoy modifying your story as your week goes along and add new and exciting details.

Practice your affirmations a minimum of twice a day. Add new ones if you can.

And keep on singing!

## DAY FIFTEEN

*<sup>18</sup> Do not remember the former things,*
*Nor consider the things of old.*
*<sup>19</sup> Behold, I will do a new thing,*
*Now it shall spring forth;*
*Shall you not know it?*
*I will even make a road in the wilderness*
*And rivers in the desert.*
Isaiah 43:18–19 (NKJV)

Dear God:

Today I celebrate that You are doing a new thing in my life! It is springing forth in my spirit and I know it! I am no longer considering the days of old when I craved unhealthy food on a regular basis. I am forgetting the former debaucheries that I labeled as a good time. As I push ahead, You are making a road for me in the wilderness of new tastes. The doubts that I had about my ability to persevere are going away because I am having the experience of rivers of water in what I thought would be a dry place of healthy eating. The roads and rivers that you have planted me on are leading to a slim body and better health! Thank you, God!

_____
_____
_____
_____
_____
_____
_____
_____
_____
_____
_____
_____
_____

## DAY SIXTEEN

*And you shall know the truth, and the*
*truth shall make you free.*
John 8:32 (NKJV)

Dear God:

Thank you for freeing me. I have been freed by the truth. The truth is that my old eating habits were being controlled by food companies that do not care about my health. Their concern for profit causes them to spend a lot of money and invest a lot time enslaving people to harm their body through excessive consumption of the wrong food. Now when I hear people say, "I am going to eat whatever I want," I realize that they are not really eating whatever they want—they are eating what someone else wants them to eat. I am free to eat the foods that I now choose to eat. I know the truth and the truth has set me free!

_____

_____

_____

_____

_____

_____

_____

_____

_____

_____

_____

_____

_____

_____

_____

_____

_____

## DAY SEVENTEEN

*Therefore if the Son makes you free, you shall be free indeed.*
John 8:36 (NKJV)

Dear God:

Thank you for all of the progress I have made! Thank you that You have been with me every step of the way! Today I know that You have been the one who set me free to take this journey. And I am indeed free through and through. I am so completely free that my mind is now beginning to imagine the other tasks that I can take on! I am excited that new and creative thoughts are in my mind. I know that I have the responsibility to share my new freedom with others in a loving way so that they too can be set free. I can't wait to see how You are going to use my testimony to break the bondage of others. I thank You, Lord, that I will be used for your glory!

_____

_____

_____

_____

_____

_____

_____

_____

_____

_____

_____

_____

_____

_____

_____

_____

_____

_____

_____

## DAY EIGHTEEN

*It is absolutely clear that God has called you to a free life.*
*Just make sure that you don't use this freedom as an excuse to*
*do whatever you want to do and destroy your freedom...*
*My counsel is this: Live freely, animated*
*and motivated by God's Spirit...*
Galatians 5:13–16 (The Message)

Dear God:

What a joy to walk in freedom! Your word says to live freely, animated and motivated by God's Spirit. I am feeling animated, free, and light today, as it has been eighteen days that I have been free from consuming excess starchy carbohydrates in my diet. I am delighted that I now have the proof that I do not need to eat carbs in excess on a daily basis. This freedom from carbs is giving me a new way of looking at the food choices I make and what I put on my plate. I know that I have the willpower to exercise portion control when I eat carbs. I am in control of me! My soul is singing the hymn, *"I am free, praise the Lord, I'm free!"*

## DAY NINETEEN

*<sup>12</sup> Not that I have already obtained all this, or have already*
*arrived at my goal, but I press on to take hold of that*
*for which Christ Jesus took hold of me.*
*<sup>13</sup> Brothers and sisters, I do not consider myself yet to have taken*
*hold of it. But one thing I do: Forgetting what is behind*
*and straining toward what is ahead,*
*<sup>14</sup> I press on toward the goal to win the prize for which God*
*has called me heavenward in Christ Jesus.*
Philippians 3:12–14 (NIV)

Dear God:

Thank you for this new day! I am greeting this day with a can-do spirit with the will and determination to keep moving forward. A famous quote says, *"You always act in a manner consistent with your innermost beliefs and convictions."* My innermost beliefs and convictions tell me that I want a slender body. I am mastering eating to be slim every day. With each new day, my new eating habits are becoming a natural part of who I am and what I believe. My innermost belief is getting stronger every day that a slender me is emerging. I am winning! I am getting closer to my goal every day!

_____
_____
_____
_____
_____
_____
_____
_____
_____
_____
_____
_____
_____

## DAY TWENTY AND TWENTY-ONE

Read over the five prayers from this week. Go back and re-read some of your favorites from weeks one and two. Record your thoughts and insights here.

_____
_____
_____
_____
_____
_____
_____
_____
_____
_____
_____
_____
_____
_____
_____
_____
_____
_____
_____
_____
_____
_____
_____
_____
_____
_____
_____
_____
_____
_____
_____

## WEEK FOUR ASSIGNMENT

Write a thank-you note from your body to yourself expressing your body's gratitude for the joyous weight loss journey you made the decision to take. The date on the note should correspond to the date on your vision board by which you have decided you will be at your ideal weight.

In the note include the different parts of your body that are thanking you. Allow your knees to thank you for the decreased stress that they feel. Maybe your mind is thanking you because it is clearer and more focused now that the excess insulin is not constantly in your system. Your arteries may be singing your praises now that bad fats have been removed from your diet and your cholesterol level has decreased. Is your face now thinner and your chin a little happier because now there is one chin where two used to be? Decreased bloating may be a benefit that has occurred because the increased fruits and vegetables in your diet are acting as a natural diuretic. As a result of the decreased bloating, your blood pressure may have dropped. Your body is now lighter and your energy may have increased. With increased energy may have come an elevation in your mood.

After your body thanks you for the wonderful changes that are occurring inside, allow you mind to thank you for what this journey has meant to you emotionally. Maybe you feel a renewed sense of confidence that is spilling over into other areas of your life. It could be that some new insights have occurred to you over the past several weeks regarding other aspects of your behavior and personality that you have decided to work on.

Let your body and mind be lavish in its praise of wonderful you. You deserve it!

Practice your affirmations every day. Add new ones if you can.

And keep on singing!

## DAY TWENTY-TWO

*[10] Finally, be strong in the Lord and in His mighty power.*
*[11] Put on the full armor of God, so that you can take*
*your stand against the devil's schemes.*
*[12] For our struggle is not against flesh and blood,*
*but against the rulers, against the authorities, against the*
*powers of this dark world and against the*
*spiritual forces of evil in the heavenly realms.*
*[13] Therefore put on the full armor of God, so that when the*
*day of evil comes, you may be able to stand your ground,*
*and after you have done everything, to stand.*
Ephesians 6:10–13 (NIV)

Dear God:

Today I am strong in the power of Your might. I recognize that while You desire the best for my life, there is an enemy that does not. I have committed to putting on Your armor every day so that I can stand my ground against any negativity that I may encounter as I embrace a healthier lifestyle. Greater are You who is in me than any spiritual force that would attempt to derail my progress. I am walking in the full authority of Your word. I can see my victory ahead of me, and by faith, I declare that it is already done!

_____

_____

_____

_____

_____

_____

_____

_____

_____

_____

## DAY TWENTY-THREE

*²⁰ My son, pay attention to what I say;*
*turn your ear to my words.*
*²¹ Do not let them out of your sight,*
*keep them within your heart;*
*²² for they are life to those who find them*
*and health to one's whole body.*
*²³ Above all else, guard your heart,*
*for everything you do flows from it.*
Proverbs 4:20–23 (NIV)

Dear God:

I bless and honor You today! It is going to be a great day! Your word tells me to guard my heart, for everything that I do flows from it. I understand that the meaning of guarding my heart is to watch what I allow my mind to experience—what I see, what I read, what I listen to, and what I meditate on. I have resolved to allow my mind to see images of me engaging in healthy behaviors of exercise, drinking water, and eating wholesome food. I have decided to read more about how to prepare a variety of healthy food. I now enjoy listening to programs about achieving good health. I meditate on the image of the slender me that I am becoming and how excited I will be when I reach my goal. Knowing that I am getting closer to my goal each day fills me with enthusiasm and joy! My heart is fully guarded from anyone and anything that would try to hinder my progress. I am on a roll like a high speed train!

_____

_____

_____

_____

_____

_____

_____

_____

## DAY TWENTY-FOUR

*Don't copy the behavior and customs of this world, but let God transform you into a new person by changing the way you think. Then you will learn to know God's will for you, which is good and pleasing and perfect.*
Romans 12:2 (NLT)

Dear God:

You are my rock and my strength! All the wisdom I will ever need to be successful in life comes from You. Your word tells me to not copy the behavior and customs of this world, but to let You transform me into a new person by changing the way that I think. I know that the behavior and customs of most people in my world are to neglect their health through poor eating habits. I have chosen to shed my past behaviors of unhealthy eating patterns for good. Through Your spirit that dwells in me, I have changed the way that I think. My thinking has been transformed so that I will now eat to be healthy and slender for life. I love how my mind has been transformed! Thank you, God!

## DAY TWENTY-FIVE

*² Why spend your money on food that does not give you strength?*
*Why pay for food that does you no good?*
*Listen to me, and you will eat what is good.*
*You will enjoy the finest food.*
*³ Come to me with your ears wide open.*
*Listen, and you will find life...*
Isaiah 55:2–3(NLT)

Dear God:

I thank you that You have supplied me with food in abundance. I am grateful that I do not lack that which I need to sustain my body. Given what I have learned about the enormous harm that processed foods can do to my body, I choose today to give heed to Your word, which tells me to eat what is good. I commit today to no longer spend my money for phony food, for food that does not build my body up, but tears it down. I choose to enjoy the finest of foods, the foods that you made. I reject foods that are so laden with chemicals that they alter my taste buds and my appreciation of what you created to sustain my life. I will delight in the abundance of good food that you have so graciously provided for me.

_____
_____
_____
_____
_____
_____
_____
_____
_____
_____
_____
_____
_____
_____

## DAY TWENTY-SIX

*¹ Make a joyful shout to the LORD, all you lands!*
*² Serve the LORD with gladness;*
*Come before His presence with singing.*
*³ Know that the LORD, He is God;*
*It is He who has made us, and not we ourselves;*
*We are His people and the sheep of His pasture.*
*⁴ Enter into His gates with thanksgiving,*
*And into His courts with praise.*
*Be thankful to Him, and bless His name.*
*⁵ For the LORD is good;*
*His mercy is everlasting,*
*And His truth endures to all generations.*
Psalms 100:1–5 (NKJV)

Dear God:

My Lord and my God, how excellent is Your name in all the earth! I have just completed almost four weeks of learning to think differently about how and what I eat. It is because of Your spirit in me that my thinking is now continuously positive und uplifting. Each new day is exciting as I see the numbers on the scale decrease. My clothes are not as snug, and that feels wonderful. I greet each new day with effervescence in my spirit! I enthusiastically choose actions that are consistent with my new perception of me in a healthy, slim body. My thoughts are my new vehicle to drive to me the destiny of being slim for life. Thank you, God, for the power you have given to me choose wise, healthy, joyous thoughts!

_____

_____

_____

_____

_____

_____

## DAY TWENTY-SEVEN AND TWENTY-EIGHT

Read over the five prayers form this week. Go back and re-read some of your favorites from the previous weeks. Record your thoughts and insights here.

_____
_____
_____
_____
_____
_____
_____
_____
_____
_____
_____
_____
_____
_____
_____
_____
_____
_____
_____
_____
_____
_____
_____
_____
_____
_____
_____
_____
_____
_____
_____

## ASSIGNMENT WEEK FIVE

It is now time to clear out some emotional clutter to keep you moving forward with a healthy mind and spirit. Grab a pen and paper and write the name of anyone whose has ever derided you about your weight. It may be that someone you love has repeatedly put you down about your weight. It could be that someone you barely knew made a cruel comment and you do not even remember his or her name, but what they said stung. Do not dwell on this exercise for long, but whatever names/situations surface within the first five minutes—these are names/ situations that you want on the list.

Once you have completed your list, give praise to God that He has released you from poor eating habits and has allowed you to enter into a new relationship with food. Thank Him also for the incredible gift of eternal life that He extended to you in John 3:16, *"For God so loved the world that He gave His only begotten Son, that whoever believes in Him should not perish but have everlasting life."* Thank Him for His promise in I John 1:9, that *"If we confess our sins, He is faithful and just to forgive us our sins and to cleanse us from all unrighteousness."* Thank Him for his word in Ephesians 4:32 which tells you, *"And be kind to one another, tenderhearted, forgiving one another, even as God in Christ forgave you."* Thank Him for His promise in Romans 8:28: *"And we know that all things work together for good to those who love God, to those who are the called according to His purpose,"* and His declaration in Romans 8:31, *"What then shall we say to these things? If God is for us, who can be against us?"*

Look at each name/situation on your list, say aloud what the person said or did that hurt you, and aloud say, "I forgive you. God has forgiven me of so much, that I now release any anger, bitterness, resentment, or hurt feelings against you. God is for me and He loves me."

It is beyond the scope of this book to do an in-depth teaching about how to let go of hurts from your past. If you need additional assistance in working through forgiving someone, email the author at info@eatyourself-slilmandneverdietagain.com and request the teaching *Making Forgiveness a Lifestyle: How to Let Go of the Baggage and Be Free.*

Practice your affirmations every day. Add new ones if you can.

And keep on singing!

## DAY TWENTY-NINE

*But those who wait on the LORD*
*Shall renew their strength;*
*They shall mount up with wings like eagles,*
*They shall run and not be weary,*
*They shall walk and not faint.*
Isaiah 40:31 (NKJV)

Dear God:

Thank you that you are renewing my strength every day. Each day I grow stronger and stronger in my resolve to eat healthy and release stored fat from my body. I started out walking down this road, and I am so delighted with all of my progress that I am ready to run to the finish line! I am mounting up with wings like eagles as my health and confidence soars! You are the wind beneath my wings! I will only go farther and higher as I continue to seek You each day for renewal and empowerment.

_____
_____
_____
_____
_____
_____
_____
_____
_____
_____
_____
_____
_____
_____
_____
_____
_____
_____
_____

## DAY THIRTY

*And God said, "See, I have given you every herb that*
*yields seed which is on the face of all the earth,*
*and every tree whose fruit yields seed;*
*to you it shall be for food."*
Genesis 1:29 (NKJV)


*And my God shall supply all your needs  according*
*to His riches in glory by Christ Jesus.*
Philippians 4:19 (NKJV)


Dear God:

Thank you, Lord, that you have provided good food for me to eat. Your earth is abundant with herbs, seeds, plants, and fruits that provide powerful nutrition to my body. I am enjoying eating more fruits and vegetables every day. I am learning more about the wonderful flavor that herbs bring to food. Thank you, God, that you truly do supply all of my needs, according to your riches in glory in Christ Jesus!

_____

_____

_____

_____

_____

_____

_____

_____

_____

_____

_____

_____

_____

_____

## DAY THIRTY-ONE

*<sup>19</sup> Or do you not know that your body is the temple*
*of the Holy Spirit who is in you, whom you have*
*from God, and you are not your own?*
*<sup>20</sup> For you were bought at a price;*
*therefore glorify God in your body*
*and in your spirit, which are God's.*
I Corinthians 19–20 (NKJV)

Dear God:

I will bless Your name at all times and Your praise shall continually be in my mouth! You are the source of my strength. You are the strength of my life. It is You who is working in me, giving me the desire and the power to do what pleases You. I know that my body is the temple of the Holy Spirit that dwells in me. My life is not my own; to you I belong. Since I belong to you, Lord, I will represent you well by my physical appearance. My appearance will be an attraction to others, rather than a distraction. When people ask me how I stay slender, I will say, "It's the God in me!"

_____
_____
_____
_____
_____
_____
_____
_____
_____
_____
_____
_____
_____
_____

## DAY THIRTY-TWO

*¹² All things are lawful for me, but all things are not helpful.*
*All things are lawful for me, but I will not be*
*brought under the power of any.*
*¹³ Foods for the stomach and the stomach for foods,*
*but God will destroy both it and them…*
I Corinthians 6: 12 – 13a (NKJV)

Dear God:

I thank you today for the freedom You have given me to choose. I celebrate that whether I choose to honor my temple with good food or not, You still love me and Your love is from everlasting to everlasting. There is no food that I can eat that will separate me from Your love. While all things are allowable for me to eat, not all foods are helpful for my body. Today I declare that I am not under the power of any food. I make wise choices every day and choose to eat foods that promote good health in my body.

_____

_____

_____

_____

_____

_____

_____

_____

_____

_____

_____

_____

_____

_____

_____

_____

## DAY THIRTY-THREE

*²³ And whatever you do, do it heartily, as to the Lord and not to men,*
*²⁴ knowing that from the Lord you will receive the reward*
*of the inheritance; for you serve the Lord Christ.*
Colossians 3:23 (NKJV)

Dear God:

In You I move, I breathe, and I have my being. My life is a precious gift from You. Thank You for giving me the mind to take care of the gift that I am. Your word tells me that whatever I do, I should do it heartily as unto You. I now eat heartily every day, knowing that I am enjoying good food that keeps my body slender and healthy. I laugh heartily because I am so delighted with all the progress I have made in just thirty-three days. I greet people heartily because I feel wonderful inside with all of the healthy changes that are occurring in my body. I am now living heartily, enjoying every moment of every day!

_____
_____
_____
_____
_____
_____
_____
_____
_____
_____
_____
_____
_____
_____
_____
_____
_____
_____

## DAY THIRTY-FOUR AND THIRTY-FIVE

Read over the five prayers from this week. Go back and re-read some of your favorites from week one to three. Record your thoughts and insights here.

_____

_____

_____

_____

_____

_____

_____

_____

_____

_____

_____

_____

_____

_____

_____

_____

_____

_____

_____

_____

_____

_____

_____

_____

_____

_____

_____

_____

_____

_____

## ASSIGNMENT WEEK SIX

You have been so successful at eating yourself slim, that you have been invited to give a talk and share your journey of weight loss. You are excited about this opportunity because you want to help others overcome bad eating habits just the way you did. Your assignment this week is to create all of the details of this talk. In creating the details, you will answer the following questions:

- Who invited you to do the talk?
- Where will the talk be held?
- Who will be in the audience?
- What's the size of the audience?
- What's the age of the audience?
- Is the audience all female, all male, or both?
- What advice you will give the audience to consider as they prepare for weight loss?
- What motivated you to eat yourself slim?
- What were some of your challenges?
- What did you find easy?
- What did you find hard?
- Who gave you support along the way?
- What was the one thing that surprised you the most during your weight loss journey?
- What helped you the most as you ate yourself slim?
- What changes do you now feel in your body?
- What lessons did you learn?
- What was the greatest benefit you experienced?
- What is your favorite new food?
- Why do you know that you will be slim for life?

Practice your affirmations every day. Add new ones if you can.

And keep on singing!

## DAY THIRTY-SIX

*37 Yet in all these things we are more than*
*conquerors through Him who loved us.*
*38 For I am persuaded that neither death nor life,*
*nor angels nor principalities nor powers,*
*nor things present nor things to come,*
*39 nor height nor depth, nor any other created thing,*
*shall be able to separate us from the love of God*
*which is in Christ Jesus our Lord.*
Romans 8:37–39 (NKJV)


Dear God:

My soul rejoices today as I think about Your goodness and mercy. I greet another day filled with possibilities and opportunities. I am more in tune to my body than I have been in a long time. With more than three-fourths of my forty-day journey to a new and slender me completed, I am so encouraged by all of my progress. Your word tells me that I am more than a conqueror through Christ Jesus. I have already conquered many bad eating habits and I profess and proclaim on this day that those habits are gone for good! The understanding of how many foods were bringing harm to my body and my brain has allowed the desire for unhealthy foods to diminish. I am enjoying new tastes and discovering new ways of enjoying foods in their natural state the way You made them to be enjoyed. Thank you for loving me so much that you gave me great food to eat!

_____

_____

_____

_____

_____

_____

_____

_____

## DAY THIRTY-SEVEN

*⁴ Delight yourself also in the LORD,*
*And He shall give you the desires of your heart.*
*⁵ Commit your way to the LORD,*
*Trust also in Him,*
*And He shall bring it to pass.*
Psalms 37:4–5 (NKJV)

Dear God:

Exceedingly great and precious promises you have given to me, oh Lord! You have promised that if I delight myself in You, You will give me the desires of my heart. The desire of my heart is that I have a slim, healthy body. As I delight myself in learning about the way You have designed nature to provide everything I need for good health, I am delighted to know that just by following your principles for eating, the desire of my heart is coming to pass! I have shed the burden on my body of eating toxic, unhealthy foods, and now have a lighter body as I delight in the foods You made in their natural state. Thank you for showing me the way!

## DAY THIRTY-EIGHT

*¹³ No temptation has overtaken you except such as
is common to man; but God is faithful, who will not allow you
to be tempted beyond what you are able,
but with the temptation will also make the way of escape,
that you may be able to bear it.*
I Corinthians 10:13 (NKJV)

Dear God:

I magnify you today and say thank you. You have been faithful to me during the past five weeks. With each temptation to give up, to turn back, to return to unhealthy habits, You have been with me. With each temptation, You have provided a way of escape. I only needed to look to You and rely on You as the source of my strength and my endurance. You are faithful. You have made new paths in my life that I can now walk down in victory. Truly I have passed from death to life, and am enjoying walking in the newness of good and vibrant health.

_____

_____

_____

_____

_____

_____

_____

_____

_____

_____

_____

_____

_____

_____

_____

_____

_____

## DAY THIRTY-NINE

*Blessed is the man who endures temptation;*
*for when he has been approved, he will receive the crown*
*of life which the Lord has promised to those who love Him.*
James 1:12 (NKJV)

Dear God:

I lift my voice today and praise Your matchless name! Through Your spirit, I have endured temptation over the past thirty-nine days and have learned to embrace the foods that you designed for me to eat. My body has shed unwanted pounds and a slender, healthier me is now my reality! The shackles of bad habits have been broken, and I will walk in victory over poor eating habits and poor health forever! I receive a crown today, and that crown has been earned because I:

> **C**: Curbed Carb Cravings
> **R**: Resisted Random Raids on the Refrigerator
> **O**: Overcame Obsessive Overeating
> **W**: Welcomed Willpower
> **N**: Neutralized Needless Nibbling

### DAY FORTY

*¹ I will extol You, my God, O King; And I will bless
Your name forever and ever.*
*² Every day I will bless You, And I will praise Your
name forever and ever.*
*³ Great is the LORD, and greatly to be praised; And
His greatness is unsearchable.*
*⁴ One generation shall praise Your works to another,
And shall declare Your mighty acts.*
*⁵ I will meditate on the glorious splendor of Your majesty,
And on Your wondrous works.*
*⁶ Men shall speak of the might of Your awesome acts,
And I will declare Your greatness.*
*⁷ They shall utter the memory of Your great goodness,
And shall sing of Your righteousness.*
*⁸ The LORD is gracious and full of compassion,
Slow to anger and great in mercy.*
*⁹ The LORD is good to all, And His tender mercies
are over all His works.*
*¹⁰ All Your works shall praise You, O LORD, And
Your saints shall bless You.*
*¹¹ They shall speak of the glory of Your kingdom,
And talk of Your power,*
*¹² To make known to the sons of men His mighty acts,
And the glorious majesty of His kingdom.*
*¹³ Your kingdom is an everlasting kingdom, And Your
dominion endures throughout all generations.*
*¹⁴ The LORD upholds all who fall, And raises up
all who are bowed down.*

*¹⁵ The eyes of all look expectantly to You, And*
*You give them their food in due season.*
*¹⁶ You open Your hand And satisfy the desire*
*of every living thing.*
*¹⁷ The LORD is righteous in all His ways,*
*Gracious in all His works.*
*¹⁸ The LORD is near to all who call upon Him,*
*To all who call upon Him in truth.*
*¹⁹ He will fulfill the desire of those who fear*
*Him; He also will hear their cry and save them.*
*²⁰ The LORD preserves all who love Him,*
*But all the wicked He will destroy.*
*²¹ My mouth shall speak the praise of the LORD,*
*And all flesh shall bless His holy name*
*Forever and ever.*
Psalm 145 (NKJV)

# CHAPTER SEVEN
## DAY FORTY-ONE AND BEYOND

Congratulations! You have completed forty days of your new eating plan and have worked to change your beliefs and mindset about food. You have removed excess fat from your body and are at or are closer to your ideal weight.

Often, losing the weight is one thing; keeping it off is another matter. You will have a huge advantage to keeping the weight off because your mind has been transformed. Remind yourself that you have been transformed for life and have no desire to return to your previous habits.

Besides enlisting the power of your new mind to keep you on track for the rest of your life, below are thirty tips to help you keep the weight off for good.

1. Continue to follow the principles that you learned in the hunter-gatherer food plan. After thirty days of your insulin secretions being reduced, you will feel so much better that you will not want to go back to the high-carb lifestyle.
2. Review the affirmations and prayers in this book. Use them to help you continue to maintain your new eating plan.
3. Educate yourself about good nutrition. The information contained in this book was to prime your pump to want to know more about what is in the food that you eat. As you educate yourself, make sure you are using reputable sources, not just something you saw on a website. I have included in the appendix a list of sources of information on the web that you can trust.

4. Educate yourself about the calorie counts in different foods. This will take a considerable amount of your time at first, but once you learn the information, it stays with you and becomes automatic.

5. Take advantage of a free calorie and fitness calculator. My Fitness Pal is a free app that you can download on your smartphone to keep track of what you are eating as you learn your new eating habits. It will also keep track of the amount of calories burn based on your exercise patterns. You will not to use this forever, just until your new eating habits become automatic.

6. Experiment with new dishes. Many of my favorite dishes are a result of recipes I found in *Cooking Light* magazine, and they have become staples of my diet.

7. Commit to eating a healthy diet that is free of trans fats and white flour. Just this commitment alone will result in your passing on a lot of dishes at parties.

8. Until you have fully transitioned into a new mindset, plan your daily eating. If you are going to be away from home where you are out and about running errands, know in advance what your food choices will be. For example, if I am shopping, I know a safe bet for me is to get a grilled KFC chicken breast (remove the skin) and a side of greens or corn. I usually get the corn because I watch the sodium in fast food, and the corn is sodium free. Besides, the corn is a starchy carb and it will make me fuller a little longer. Other safe bets are McDonald's grilled chicken salads; just skip the dressings or use a small amount of the low-fat dressings. Salads with dressings are usually high in fat and sodium. If you are hankering for a sandwich, Chik-Fil-A grilled chicken on wheat bread is a safe bet; just use mustard as your condiment, and try eating only one side of the bun to cut down on the carbs. You can download a fast food nutrition application for your smart phone so you can have the nutritional information readily available.

9. Monitor portion size. As you begin to change your eating habits, use measuring cups and spoons so you get an idea of what exactly what one tablespoon of sour cream or a one-half cup of rice looks like. When most people eat pasta, they really are eating 3–4 servings.

10. Eat until you are no longer hungry, not until you are full. Maybe once or twice a year, I eat until I feel full. Whether it is Thanksgiving dinner or dining at my favorite restaurant, I never eat until I feel full. I

always leave the table with room in my stomach for more food if the situation presented itself and it was something that I wanted to taste.

11. Learn to dine, not just eat. Dining is a different experience from eating. Dining connotes a relaxing time of pleasure and enjoyment when eating. Eating, on the other hand, is something we do at our desk, in our car, or on the run. People who take the time to dine are more conscious of what they eat and they tend to eat less.

12. Weigh yourself once a week. Research suggests that people who keep an eye on the number on the scale tend to keep the weight off that they lose. This will avoid weight creep. You should weigh yourself on the same day of the week at the same time of day. I weigh myself every Friday, first thing in the morning before I eat or drink anything, sans pajamas.

13. If you experience weight creep, stop it at two or three pounds. It is unsafe to practice a ten-pound weight swing. This will lead to yo-yo dieting, which can cause you to lose lean muscle and increase the percentage of fat on your body. Commit to taking off any excess weight immediately. Two pounds can turn into four, and then four can turn into eight. You can return to the beginning phase of the weight loss plan and lose the weight quickly.

14. Get enough rest. When you are not getting enough sleep, your body will produce greater quantities of the hormone ghrelin, which stimulates your appetite, while at the same it will produce a lesser quantity of the hormone leptin, which tells you when you are full.

15. Drink at least 64 ounces of water a day. Water helps to keep you feeling full and helps you to eat less. It is reported that many people confuse being thirsty with being hungry, so rather than quench their thirst with calorie-free water, they eat.

16. Always eat breakfast. When you sleep, your metabolism slows down. Eating breakfast wakes it back up again and helps your body to begin burning calories more efficiently.

17. Eat throughout the day. Having frequent small meals is preferable to having just two or three large meals. I eat six times a day. Breakfast, snack, lunch, snack, dinner, snack. My snacks are preplanned and I carry them with me wherever I go so I will not be caught off guard and head to the vending machine. At home, my favorite snack is Greek yogurt, low-fat cheddar cheese, or nuts. On the go, my favorite snack is almonds or walnuts.

18. Eat most of your carbs early in the day. A good plan is to not eat carbs past 6:00 p.m. If you get a craving for a late snack, eat lean protein.

19. Enjoy your favorite food. Whatever your favorite food is, learn to enjoy it occasionally as part of your new healthy eating plan. I must warn you, once you educate yourself about food, some of your favorite foods may not be your favorites anymore. This happened to me with chicken wings. Do you remember when McDonald's sold Mighty Wings? I was hooked! I can still recall with clarity the day when I went to McDonald's to order them, only to find out they had been discontinued from the menu. I was both grief stricken and bewildered, and had to go to my car to regain my composure! However, once I understood that eating poultry skin, especially after it had been fried, was contradictory to good health in a major way, I no longer wanted to eat chicken wings of any kind. Everyone has something that she just can't imagine never eating again, so whatever it is for you, give yourself permission to eat and fit it into your food and exercise plan. My one food that is with me for life is chocolate. I just can't imagine not eating it regularly.

20. Only keep food in the house that is part of your healthy eating plan. Tempting yourself by having cookies and chips on hand is a no-no.

21. Know your trouble spots. Determine which settings cause you to overeat and plan for these occasions. You can plan by reducing your calories a few days before so you create a calorie deficit, and then have a work-out strategy for the day(s) following the over-indulgence.

22. Have a vacation eating plan. Vacations are a trouble spot for most people, especially if you like to take cruises. Remind yourself that you are on vacation for the relaxation, the fun, and the sightseeing, not to gain weight. For seven- to ten-day vacations, I have a vacation eating plan that allows me to gain no more than one pound. I stick to eating my normal breakfast and lunch, and will splurge a little on some dinners. I also increase the intensity and the duration of my workouts to compensate for the extra food that I might eat.

23. When you are in social settings, rather than munch on the familiar dips, chips, cheese, crackers, etc., save your calories for something that you really want to eat and enjoy, or to try something new. Teach yourself that social functions are for you to socialize, not to go and eat every hors d'oeuvre you see. Eat a light meal before you go, so you

won't get to the event and be ravenous. Learn to pass up the high-carb, high-fat, high-sugar snacks.

24. At big holiday dinners, eat your favorite foods, not everything that is served. This is the strategy that I use at Thanksgiving and Christmas dinner. Our family serves a smorgasbord at these meals. What I look forward to on Thanksgiving and Christmas is a dinner with turkey, cranberry sauce, dressing, gravy, and an old-fashioned dinner roll. With the exception of the turkey, I do not normally eat these foods at any other time of the year. So these are the foods that I put on my plate. The rest of the foods I easily pass up, or I may taste a tablespoon of them. But for the most part, I can get them any time, so I do not eat them at the holiday dinner.

25. Exercise must be a regular part of your new lifestyle. Find fun and exciting ways to exercise like learning kickboxing, belly dancing, or ballroom dancing. Line dancing is popular and is offered through local parks and recreation sites at a nominal fee. If you have cable TV, experiment with the many exercise programs that are offered free of charge.

26. Get rid of the clothes that are too big for you. Holding on to pants that are too large just in case you gain weight only gives you permission to gain weight. Every item of clothing in your closet should be something that can fit you and fit you well. If they do not fit you, they are somebody else's clothes.

27. Remember that the days of your being inactive and overweight were not the good old days; you were not happy with your body then. Do not dwell on the food you used to be able to eat without gaining an ounce. That time is past and you have adjusted your calories and your activity level to keep your body at a size with which you are pleased.

28. Implement the discipline of fasting from food in your life. Fasting gives you great discipline to turn away unhealthy foods. Begin by fasting from noon to noon. I like this type of fast because on day one, you will eat breakfast and lunch. You skip dinner, and rather than food, you drink herbal tea sweetened with a natural sweetener or diluted fruit juice. Fresh juice that you make with your own juicer is best. You will skip breakfast the next morning, then re-introduce food again at lunch. Work your way to a full-day fast where you sip only tea sweetened with natural sweeteners or diluted fruit juice. I

recommend that you try fasting once a month on a day where you do not have a lot of activities planned.

29. Once you reach your ideal weight, take a picture and post it along with a picture of you before your weight loss. Post this picture where you can see it daily as a reminder of why you have adopted your new healthy eating plan.

30. Lighten up and forgive yourself! You will not be perfect as you adjust to a new eating and exercise lifestyle. Let go of any guilt you may experience by eating something decadent or skipping exercise for a few days. Keep your life in balance.

# Epilogue
## VICTORY

*Victory! Oh, how sweet the sound!*
*And the changes I've made, even more profound.*
*The promise was that if I heeded the advice in this book,*
*I would have a new mind and body—and I got it, just look!*
*Not bragging, just saying, "I'm looking good and I know it!"*
*A new body has emerged and I'm not afraid to flaunt it.*
*I am hooked on a new and healthy lifestyle,*
*I exercise regularly and can walk for miles.*
*Free from food foibles (the alliteration is cute),*
*With the knowledge I have gained I am now very astute.*
*I make wise choices when I sit down to eat and drink,*
*It is now automatic and I don't even have to think!*
*Shopping for and preparing healthy dishes is now a way of life,*
*It happens naturally without any grief or strife.*
*No longer about self-control, starvation, or denying myself,*
*I desire food that is good for my body and protects my health.*
*It is a joy to eat food that is both tasty and good for me,*
*I am living proof that anyone can gain the victory!*

# APPENDIX

## NATURAL WEIGHT LOSS SUPPLEMENTS

Whether or not you choose to supplement your weight loss efforts with a pill is entirely your decision. I am including this section so you will know what the current trends are in reportedly safe and close to natural supplements. I encourage you to research any supplement that you may decide to take using resources such as the International Journal of Obesity, American Journal of Clinical Nutrition, National Institutes of Health, New England Journal of Medicine, Mayo Clinic, etc. (this just might be my next book!) Any website that is providing information while also trying to sell you a product should not be trusted as a reliable source of information.

There are numerous weight loss supplements with acceptable research as to their effectiveness. The challenge becomes in finding a brand of the supplement that delivers the results shown in research studies. While the pharmaceutical industry is highly regulated and it can take years to get a new drug on the market, the supplement industry is highly unregulated. The purity, safety or effectiveness of any product cannot be guaranteed unless the manufacturer has completed scientifically valid research on their own product using an independent agent or lab. Supplement manufacturers overwhelmingly use "borrowed research" to sell their product. They will say in their advertisement that studies show that XYZ helps to burn belly fat. This will be a true statement. But what they do not say and cannot say is whether or not their particular product with its unique formulation has been proven to do the same thing.

With the above in mind, the supplements listed here may be helpful. I have not tried any of these supplements so I cannot personally endorse them.

Adiponectin:   A protein hormone produced and secreted  by fat cells that regulates the metabolism of fat and glucose.   Low levels of adiponectin are found in people who are obese.   Numerous weight loss supplements are now including this hormone in their formulation.

African Mango : The African Mango diet is the newest diet/supplement on the market promising rapid weight loss by eliminating unwanted fats from the body. Eating a specific wild mango from Cameroon Africa is supposed to help lower cholesterol and drop the pounds due to the active component Irvingia Gabonensis (IGOB131). The extract is found in the seed not the fruit pulp itself and most people do not eat the seed. There are very few studies to date on IGOB131 and weight loss. More studies are required to conclude that IGOB131 is effective for weight loss in humans.   http:// www.sharecare.com/question/what-african-mango-diet.

Capsaicin: Capsaicin is a natural compound in chili peppers. It is said to boost metabolism, decrease appetite, and reduce fat. Some preliminary studies suggest that this spicy chemical may be of some benefit to those trying to slim down.

Fucoxanthin:  This compound was discussed in the text as a metabolism booster and can be derived by making a broth. It is also available as a nutritional supplement in capsule form and can be found in some health food stores and online.

Green Coffee Beans: Green coffee refers to coffee in its rawest, purest form. The unroasted seeds, or beans, of coffee fruits may slow glucose absorption and stop fat from accumulating all over your body. In a new study, participants who took the supplement did not exercise nor did they change their diet, yet they lost over 10% of their body weight on average. To benefit from green coffee bean extract, take 800 mg twice a day about 30 minutes before breakfast and dinner with a large glass of water. Be sure to purchase "pure" green coffee bean extract, free of binders, cellulose, or other additives. http://www.sharecare.com/question/how-green-coffee-extract-lose-weight.

Raspberry Ketones:  Raspberry ketones, a natural compound found in red raspberries, helps your body to burn fat by breaking up fats within your cells. It contains the hormone adiponectin that boosts metabolism. The supplement is recommended because you'd have to eat 90 pounds of raspberries to get the same effect. Take 100 milligrams of raspberry ketone at breakfast time. http://www.sharecare.com/question/lose-body-fat.

White Bean Extract:  White bean extract blocks starch and prevents carbs from being absorbed in the body. Studies show if you absorb fewer calories, you'll lose fat and your metabolism will speed up. Take one tablet each day before a meal. http://www.sharecare.com/question/what-are-inexpensive-metabolism-boosters.

## TRUSTED SOURCES OF INFORMATION ON THE INTERNET

As you desire to grow in your knowledge about good nutrition, be wary of what you read on the internet. Many sources of information have an ulterior motive and that is to sell you something. There is so much misinformation online and thousands of people are proclaiming that they have the truth.

There is often a disagreement between traditional medicine and alternative health practitioners. Alternative medicine is sometimes ahead of the curve when it comes to nutrition information. If there is a difference of opinion, I always lean more toward the one from the alternative medical professional.

I recommend the following websites from which you can feel confident that information is accurate.

*Traditional Medicine*

Mayo Clinic: www.mayoclinic.com

Sharecare: www.sharecare.com

National Institutes of Health: nih.com

Centers for Disease Control: cdc.gov

WebMD: www.webmd.com

*Alternative Medicine*

About.com: www.about.com  The information contained on about.com references reputable journal articles in their discussion of alternative health practices.

Andrew Weil: www.drweil.com.  Dr. Weil's training in traditional medicine makes his knowledge base sound and a good platform for understanding medical issues. Just a note: this site contains a lot of products for sale. Be discerning when ordering.

## Recommended Reading on Nutrition and Natural Health

*The Maker's Diet* by Rubin Jordan, Ph.D.  Siloam a Strang Company

*From Here to Longevity* by Mitra Ray, Ph.D.  Shining Star Publishing

*Empty Harvest* by Bernard Jensen, DCM & Mark Anderson.
Avery/Penguin Putnam, Inc.

*Fats that Heal, Fats that Kill.* Udo Erasmus.  Alive Publishing Group

*Your Miracle Brain* by Jean Carper.  Harper-Collins Publisher

*The Omega-3 Connection* by Andrew L. Stoll, M.D. Simon & Schuster Publishers

# ABOUT THE AUTHOR

Etrulia Reid "Troy" Lee (Dr. Troy) is a native of Philadelphia, Pennsylvania. She has resided in the Washington, D.C., metro area since 1978, and currently makes her home in Fort Washington, Maryland, where she lives with her husband, Arvid Lee. She has two adult sons, Chay and Michael.

Dr. Troy has been in the field of education for over thirty years. She completed her undergraduate work in education at Cabrini College in Radnor, Pennsylvania, and her master's degree at the University of Maryland in College Park, also in education. She completed her Ph.D. in holistic nutrition at Clayton College of Natural Health in Birmingham, Alabama.

Dr. Troy began her career as a classroom teacher, and has held various positions in the education field, such as coordinator for a day care for disabled preschoolers, consultant to group homes for physically and mentally disabled children and adults, instructor at the USDA graduate school, school principal, education division superintendent for a Christian ministry, author, and speaker. She is an adjunct professor at Global Health College, where she teaches nutrition.

An interest in healthy eating and weight control were topics that interested Dr. Troy for many years. It was in her role as school principal in 1998 that her interest turned into a passion. It was there that she discovered that an alarming percentage of children had allergies and asthma and that these conditions were due in part to children being born with compromised immune systems. Research suggested that this was as a result of poor nutrition during pregnancy, despite the fact that the mothers followed the recommended nutritional guidelines and took prenatal vitamins. The quality of the standard American diet was so poor that it put children at

.sk. This inspired her to learn more about nutrition so she could share this information with parents.

Dr. Troy challenges her audiences to evaluate how their lifestyle and diet are contributing to the many illnesses they may have, and how it puts them at risk for future disease and premature death. She offers personal coaching and facilitates support groups for people wanting to change their eating habits.

In addition to championing weight loss, Dr. Troy is a sought-after speaker and provides fun, interactive workshops on several topics which are listed below. All of the workshops below are also available on CD.

- How to Write a Personal Mission Statement to Achieve Your Destiny
- The Principles and Power of Goal Setting: How to Create an Action Plan to Achieve Your Goals
- Conflict Resolution in the Workplace
- Making Forgiveness a Lifestyle: How to Let Go of the Baggage and Be Free
- What Every Parent Should Know About How the Brain Develops
- Nutrition and Learning
- Healthy Lifestyles: Nutrition, Stress Reduction, and Exercise
- Are You Losing Your Mind? How Different Foods Affect the Structure and Function of the Brain
- Is Your Body on Fire? Understanding Inflammation: The Number One Cause of Sickness and Disease

Dr. Troy would love to hear from you and the progress you have made on your journey to be slim for life. You may email her at info@eatyourself-slimandneverdietagain.com or leave a comment on her Facebook page at How to Eat Yourself Slim and Never Diet Again. You may also contact her via mail at P.O. Box 44086, 11550 Livingston Road, Fort Washington, MD 20749.

You may also want to join the fun online with the Eat Yourself Slim and Never Diet Again boot camps. The six -week boot camps are powerful, energizing, and motivating to help you shake the weight for good! Designed to parallel your journey as you read this book, online sessions allow you to interact live with Dr. Troy every week, receive coaching, and pair up with an accountability partner. You may register at www.eatslimtoday.com or www.eatyourslimandneverdietagain.com.